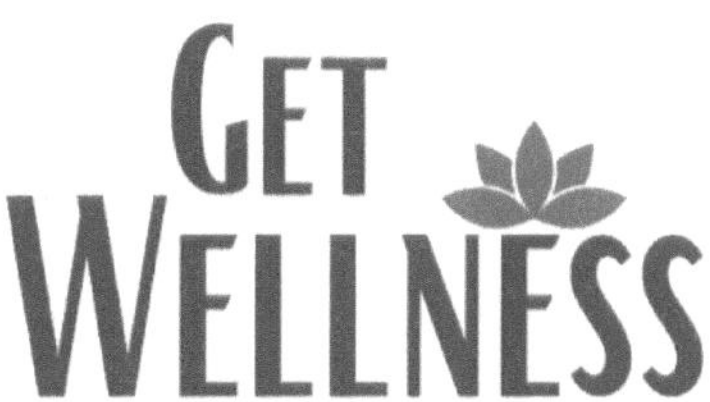

GET WELLNESS

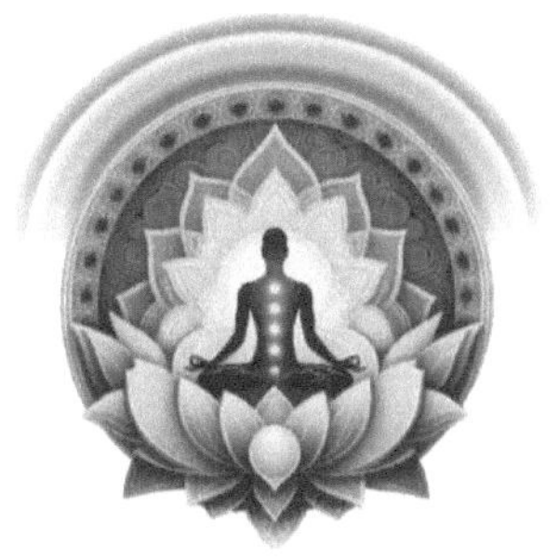

Embrace Holistic Healing, Blend Ancient Wisdom with Modern Science, Unleash your wellness, and Rediscover the Joy of Living.

By

Dr. Prakash Shah

Email: prakashbaroda45@gmail.com

Website: www.chronictreat.com

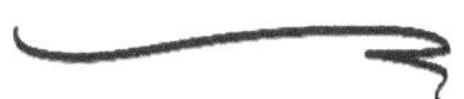

WHY IS THIS BOOK FOR YOU?

"Get Wellness" offers invaluable insights garnered from **Dr. Prakash Shah's** half-century of medical practice, revealing the profound yet simple knowledge essential for disease prevention and management.

In a world where minor oversights often lead to severe health consequences, this book serves as a beacon of guidance, empowering readers with the fundamental principles necessary to safeguard their well-being.

Through the lens of homeostasis, the body's innate balancing mechanism, Dr. Shah illustrates how birds and animals effortlessly maintain their health, a testament to the efficacy of natural mechanisms. Drawing on examples from cultures like Japan and China, where longevity is revered, Dr. Shah underscores the importance of understanding and adhering to these foundational principles. This book isn't just for adults—it's a vital resource that should be placed in the hands of every child, fostering a culture of health literacy from a young age.

By instilling basic knowledge, behaviors, and habits conducive to wellness, **"Get Wellness"** empowers individuals to take charge of their health, ultimately benefiting society as a whole. Dr. Shah eloquently compares the body to a well-managed factory, where each department works harmoniously under the supervision of the owner and manager—our innate biological mechanisms.

Through simple yet profound insights, readers learn that maintaining good health isn't complex; it's a matter of adhering to straightforward guidelines and principles.

With **"Get Wellness,"** readers gain not only knowledge but also the tools to lead vibrant, healthy lives. By embracing the wisdom within these pages, individuals can unlock the secrets to longevity and vitality, steering clear of preventable illnesses and enjoying the boundless benefits of a robust mind-body connection.

Dr. Shah's holistic approach emphasizes the importance of integrating various treatment modalities, from allopathy to homeopathy and Ayurveda, highlighting the multifaceted nature of health management.

Backed by thorough research and international expertise, **"Get Wellness"** is a comprehensive guide that equips readers with the essential knowledge and practices needed to cultivate lasting well-being.

TABLE OF CONTENTS

INTRODUCTION 7

METHODS OF TREATMENT 11

BIOLOGY OF DISEASES 31

CONVENTIONAL VS. ALTERNATIVE MEDICINES 35

CHRONIC DISEASES UNDERSTANDING 49

ALLOPATHIC MEDICINES 57

DEFINITION OF ALLOPATHIC MEDICINE 73

ALLOPATHIC MEDICINES 79

AYURVEDIC SYSTEM 87

HOMEOPATHY 109

STRESS 125

DISCLAIMER 131

ABOUT ME...133

MAY I ASK YOU FOR A SMALL FAVOR? 139

INTRODUCTION

In my 50 years of medical practice, I have found that most people do not have simple knowledge for avoiding diseases, and by very small misunderstanding, they suffer from grave diseases. Then they spend valuable money, and even then, they go on suffering. Very learned and high-class people make small mistakes. If they had even basic knowledge, they would not have suffered so much, and lots of money- time and suffering would have been saved. From very small mistakes, major diseases enter the body that produce more severe diseases.

I have prepared this book to give general knowledge for avoiding and curing diseases. God has endowed everybody with a coordinating mechanism known as homeostasis. Birds and animals adhere to these mechanisms, ensuring their sustained health throughout their lifetimes, succumbing only at life's end. They adeptly maintain bodily functions. In countries like Japan and China, certain tribes have achieved lifespans exceeding 100 years.

This book should be presented to every younger child individually, and all children should be encouraged to read again and again when time permits. This will encourage them to have the basic knowledge, behavior, and habits to become healthy citizens, which will be a great advantage to the country. This basic knowledge encourages everyone to stay healthy. Health is everyone's concern.

Our body is like a factory with many departments. Each department is a separate entity, but they work in harmony to achieve the best outcome. All departments have very good connections and coordination. The manager and owner supervise to achieve harmony.

If people understand a few basic principles of health, they will have great benefits. Healthy life and healthy living. Health is wealth. To remain healthy, everyone has to follow very easy and very simple guidelines.

For healthy living, we have to follow simple rules, and that will give us a healthy life with the passion of a healthy mind and a healthy body.

There are many methods to treat diseases. Methods for keeping a healthy body must be learned.

By simply reading this book, everyone will have knowledge that is advantageous to the body and that can avoid ill effects and diseases in the body. This is the knowledge everyone is required to have. Simple care can avoid many diseases and produce healthy living. Simple and small care of the body will go a long way to having good health. So, methods for maintaining a normal body need to be known and practiced. All precautions and more research and knowledge are required.

Allopathy, Homeopathy, and Ayurveda are the primary systems of treatment practiced today, although numerous other treatment modalities exist. When discussing a particular topic, it may be necessary to acknowledge these other systems, as their mention is relevant.

Help and citations are taken from books, literature, and international search engines. I am thankful for their liberty.

I pray that God will make everyone's life healthy.

In my medical practice, I am consistently prepared to assist patients who are unwell and suffering. Integrating alternative medicines and offering straightforward guidance can sometimes yield miraculous results. Witnessing my patients achieve full recovery brings me immense joy. I am always reachable via email at prakashbaroda45@gmail.com

METHODS OF TREATMENT

Drugs, surgeries, procedures, and vaccines are the main ways in which medical doctors and scientists treat diseases. Drug treatments include antibiotics, which are used to cure bacterial diseases, as well as anti-inflammatory medications and water pills.

Diagnosis

Your doctor may order lab work or imaging scans to help determine what's causing your symptoms.

Treatment

Knowing what type of germ is causing your illness makes it easier for your doctor to choose the appropriate treatment.

Antibiotics

Antibiotics are grouped into "families" of similar types. Bacteria are also put together in groups of similar types, such as streptococcus or E. coli.

Certain types of bacteria are especially susceptible to particular classes of antibiotics. If your doctor knows what type of bacteria you're infected with, treatment can be targeted more precisely.

Antibiotics are usually reserved for bacterial infections because they do not affect illnesses caused by viruses. But sometimes, it's difficult to tell which type of germ is at work.

For example, pneumonia can be caused by a bacterium, a virus, a fungus, or a parasite. The overuse of antibiotics has resulted in several types of bacteria developing resistance to one or more varieties of antibiotics, making these bacteria much more difficult to treat.

Antivirals

Drugs have been developed to treat some, but not all, viruses. Examples include the viruses that cause:

- HIV/AIDS

- Herpes

- Hepatitis B

- Hepatitis C

- Influenza

Antifungals

Topical antifungal medications can be used to treat skin or nail infections caused by fungi. Some fungal infections, such as those affecting the lungs or the mucous membranes, can be treated with an oral antifungal. More severe internal organ fungal infections, especially in people with weakened immune systems, may require intravenous antifungal medications.

Anti-parasitics

Some diseases, including malaria, are caused by tiny parasites. While there are drugs to treat these diseases, some varieties of parasites have developed resistance to the drugs.

Some of the substances that have been studied for preventing or shortening the duration of infection include:

- Cranberry

- Echinacea

- Garlic

- Ginseng

- Goldenseal

- Vitamin C

- Vitamin D

- Zinc

Preparing for your appointment

You'll probably first see your primary care doctor. Depending on the severity of your infection, as well as which of your organ systems is affected by the infection, your doctor may refer you to a specialist. For example, a dermatologist specializes in skin conditions and a pulmonologist treats lung disorders.

What you can do

You may want to write a list that includes:

- Detailed descriptions of your symptoms

- Information about medical problems you've had

- Information about your parents' or siblings' medical problems

- All the medications and dietary supplements you take

- Questions you want to ask the doctor

Preparing a list of questions for your doctor will help you make the most of your time together. For infectious diseases, some basic questions to ask your doctor include:

- What's the most likely cause of my symptoms?

- Are there other possible causes for my symptoms?

- What kinds of tests do I need?

- Is my condition likely temporary or long-lasting?

- What treatment do you recommend?

- I have other health conditions. How can I best manage these conditions together?

- Is there a generic alternative to the medicine you're prescribing?

- Are there any brochures or other printed material that I can take home with me? What websites do you recommend?

What to expect from your doctor

Your doctor is likely to ask you a number of questions, including:

- When did your symptoms begin?

- Do your symptoms come and go, or do you have symptoms all the time?

- How severe are your symptoms?

- Have you recently come into contact with anyone who's sick?

- Have you been bitten or scratched by an animal or come into contact with animal feces?

- Do you have any insect bites?

- Have you eaten undercooked meat or unwashed vegetables?

- Have you been out of the country recently?

— Being **cured** of a **disease** means it's completely gone and isn't coming back. For many people, **cures** represent the ultimate treatment goal.

ANSWER

Before trying to cure a disease, the first question a scientist would ask is, "What's causing the disease?" We would normally start by figuring out what part of the body is most affected by the disease and then figure out what changes in the diseased or sick tissue.

For example, cancer cells usually grow much faster than normal cells, and that can be caused by many different kinds of proteins that affect how a cell grows and divides. Scientists now have a panel of "likely suspects" in this case, and we test tumor samples for those protein suspects using a variety of means. Once the cause of the change in the diseased cell or tissue has been identified, the search for a cure can begin. Sometimes, the cause is the lack of a protein or the fact that an altered version of the protein is produced, like in sickle cell anemia with hemoglobin. One way that scientists cure a disease, in this case, is to give back the good protein to the cells in the form of the DNA or gene for this protein. This so-called gene therapy is still pretty new, but scientists like myself think the future of this method of curing a disease has some great potential.

Other times, the cause of the disease is that the new protein acts differently than the normal one. It might be that the protein can interact with proteins or other molecules that it would not normally "hang out" with.

Other times, the cause of the disease is that the new protein acts differently than the normal one. It might be that the protein can interact with proteins or other molecules that it would not normally "hang out" with.

Developing drugs that act on the "sick" protein and do not affect any other normal or good process in the human body can be a long process. Once these drugs are found and developed, they can often help scientists better understand and treat diseases in many people.

Infectious disease may be an unavoidable fact of life. Still, there are many strategies available to help

us protect ourselves from infection and treat disease once it has developed.

Vaccines and Medicines

Medicines have existed in human society probably as long as the sickness itself. However, with the advent of the modern pharmaceutical industry, biochemical approaches to preventing and treating disease have acquired a new level of prominence in the evolving relationship between microbes and their human hosts.

Antibiotics are powerful medicines that fight bacterial infections. They either kill bacteria or stop them from reproducing, allowing the body's natural defenses to eliminate the pathogens. Used properly, antibiotics can save lives. However, growing antibiotic resistance is curbing the effectiveness of these drugs. Taking an antibiotic as directed, even after symptoms disappear, is key to curing an infection and preventing the development of resistant bacteria.

Antibiotics don't work against viral infections such as colds or the flu.

Antiviral drugs are now available to treat a number of viruses, including influenza, HIV, herpes, and hepatitis B. Like bacteria, viruses mutate over time and develop resistance to antiviral drugs

Modern medicine needs new kinds of antibiotics and antivirals to treat drug-resistant infections

New antiviral drugs are also in short supply. These medicines have been much more difficult to develop than antibacterial drugs because antivirals can damage host cells where the viruses reside.

which provides an integrated, systematic approach to the development and purchase of the vaccines, drugs, therapies, and diagnostic tools necessary for public health medical emergencies

Daily habits provide some of the strongest defenses against infectious diseases. Among the sensible actions you can take:

- **Keep immunizations up to date**

Wash your hands often. Washing with regular soap and rinsing with running water, followed by thorough drying, is considered the most important way to prevent disease transmission. Routine consumer use of

Use antibiotics only for infections caused by bacteria. Viral infections cannot be treated with antibiotics.

- **Report to your doctor any rapidly worsening infection or any infection that does not get better after taking a course of antibiotics, if prescribed.**

Stay alert to disease threats when traveling or visiting underdeveloped countries.

- **Acquire healthy habits such as eating well, getting enough sleep, exercising, and avoiding tobacco and illegal drug use.**

Foodborne diseases are largely preventable—but the goal requires vigilance in every step from the farm to the table.

Technological advances in disease surveillance and detection, such as regional syndromic surveillance, bioinformatics, and rapid diagnostic methods, have strengthened infectious disease control and prevention efforts.

By identifying viruses, bacteria, and parasites in animals where they naturally live and monitoring those organisms as they move from animals into people, it may be possible to prevent deadly new infections of animal origin from entering and racing through human populations.

Microorganisms are our friends and foes. Some of them are useful for us, while some of them are harmful.

An antibiotic is a chemical substance that inhibits the growth of bacteria. It hinders the reproductive cycle of the bacteria inside the host's body.

Lactobacillus is a genus of bacteria that can convert sugars into lactic acid by means of fermentation.

A vaccine is a biological preparation that provides active acquired immunity to a particular disease. It has killed or weakened the suspension of microorganisms, which generates the immune response.

What was directly responsible for the rapid rise of the world population in the twentieth century?

a) Increased food production

b)   Better transport facilities

c)   Better education and job prospects

d)   Use of antibiotics and prophylactic vaccinations

What is Health?

The World Health Organisation (WHO) gave the following definition of health in 1948. "Health is a state of complete physical, mental and social well-being and not merely the absence of disease or infirmity." The WHO definition of health recognizes three dimensions of health, i.e., physical, mental, and social. In 1978, another thing was included in this definition. It is the ability to lead a "Socially and economically productive life."

It is rightly said that Health is Wealth. There are various factors which influence health. These factors lie both within the individual and also in the society in which they live. The internal factors are basically the genetic makeup of an individual, while external factors lie in the environment to which they are exposed.

Personal health is a state of complete physical, mental, and social well-being. Community health comprises maintaining, improving, and protecting the health of the entire community. The various factors that help in maintaining community health are:

- Maintaining proper hygienic and sanitary conditions of the environment.

- Providing good socio-economic conditions.

- Providing health care services.

- Imparting health education and promoting public awareness.

- Providing proper facilities for preventing diseases.

Basic Conditions for Good Health

'A sound mind in a sound body' is an old saying and expresses the importance of good health.

Distinctions between Healthy and Disease-free

Too often, we confuse being healthy with being disease-free. However, it is not the same thing at all! There are many differences between the two. Below, we will look at the basic differences between the two.

Disease-free	Healthy
One who is not suffering from any disease or derangement of the functioning of the body.	Health is a state of physical, mental, and social well-being.
It refers to the individual.	It refers not only to the individual but also to the social and community environment.
A disease-free individual may have good health or poor health	A healthy individual is able to perform normally in a given situation.

Principles of Treatment

The immune system is a major factor that determines the number of microbes surviving in the body. There are two ways to treat an infectious disease, i.e.,

- To reduce the effects of the disease

- To kill the cause of the disease

In the first case, treatment reduces the symptoms due to inflammation. A doctor gives medicine to the patient to bring down the fever and reduce pain or loose motions. One must also rest in bed so that one can conserve energy, enabling one to have more energy to focus on healing.

How do the Medicines Work?

To cure the disease, the microbes have to be killed by the use of medicine. As you know, we can classify microbes into different categories. They are viruses, bacteria, fungi, or protozoa. Each of these groups of organisms will have some essential biochemical life processes that are peculiar to that group and are not shared with the other groups.

These processes may be pathways for the synthesis of new substances or respiration. For example, our cells may make new substances by a mechanism different from that used by bacteria. Therefore, a drug that can block the bacterial synthesis pathway without affecting our own is used to cure a bacterial disease. Antibiotic drugs work on the same principle. Similarly, some drugs, such as malarial parasites, kill protozoa without affecting our bodies.

Viruses have only a few biochemical mechanisms of their own. This is the reason why making antiviral medicines is more difficult than making antibacterial medicines. The viruses enter the host cells and use the host's machinery for their life processes. Therefore, there are relatively few virus drugs that check a number of viral diseases, including HIV infection.

Prevention of Diseases

There are two ways to prevent diseases.

- General

- Specific to a disease

In general, we can prevent exposure to diseases by providing good living conditions, such as drinking safe water and having a clean environment. In specific prevention, the immune system in our body normally fights off microbes. Our cells specialize in killing infecting microbes.

These cells go into action when microbes enter into the body. The immune cells manage to kill off the infection long before it assumes major proportions. The immune system will function well if proper and sufficient nourishment and food are available. There are also some specific ways to prevent infections, like vaccination for a particular disease.

But what, exactly, is suffering? One patient with cancer of the stomach, from which he knew he would shortly die, said he was not suffering. Another, someone who had been operated on for a minor problem—in little pain and not seemingly distressed—said that even coming into the hospital had been a source of pain and suffering. With such varied responses to the problem of suffering, inevitable questions arise. Is it the doctor's responsibility to treat the disease or the patient? And what is the relationship between suffering and the goals of medicine?

Ideas in Conflict: The Rise and Fall of New Views of Disease

discusses the changing concept of the ideal physician. It begins by presenting four points in relation to the changes in the character of physicians before moving on to discussing the effects of science on the ideal of the doctor, the impact of technology as distinct from science, and the changes in the doctor-patient relationship. The chapter also looks at the increasing interest in medical ethics and the concept of commercialism.

Suffering and its nature have been given little attention despite the fact that physicians are obligated to relieve human suffering. The majority of the chapter discusses three main points: suffering is experienced by persons, suffering occurs when the impending destruction of a person is perceived, and suffering can occur in relation to any aspect of a person.

Suffering from Chronic Illness

This chapter discusses suffering from chronic illness. It starts with a definition of chronic illness and its symptoms. The chapter discusses one of the alterations produced by chronic illness, which is a changing perception of the world, and also presents several strategies for reducing suffering.

This chapter discusses the relationship between doctor and patient. This refers to the central and basic relationship between doctor and patient that rests solely on the fact that one is a patient and the other is a doctor. The chapter looks at the physician as a person, what defines a good physician, and the relation between trust and altruism. The final portion of the chapter centers on self-discipline, which is necessary not only for thoroughness but also for the maintenance of knowledge, patient consistency, and nerves.

The Mysterious Relationship Between Doctor and Patient

- The Physician as a Person

- What Defines a Good Physician

- The Relation Between Trust and Altruism

- Self-Discipline

This chapter discusses and addresses the difficult issues that must be faced and solved before shifting the primary concern from diseases to a focus on sick persons. It shows why disease theory has been so necessary and successful for clinicians or the doctors who actually take care of the patients. The chapter then looks at three common diseases to show how the ideas contained in classic disease theory are exemplified and used in the practice of medicine. It also illustrates the practical consequences of the changes that have taken place in the axioms of disease theory over the last few decades.

This chapter discusses the relationship between the sick person and the sickness and between the disease entity and its existence in a sick person. It examines the place of symptoms in medical care and how these symptoms become symptoms for the patient. The chapter looks at the relationship of a symptom to suffering and determines which is real: symptoms or diseases.

The Pursuit of Disease or the Care of the Sick?

- "Doctor, What Is Wrong with Me?"

- How Symptoms Get to Be Symptoms for the Patient

- The Relationship of a Symptom to Suffering

- Which Is Real, Symptoms or Diseases?

- Who Puts Humpty Dumpty Back Together Again?

- "Have You Found the Cause of My ..."

- An Illness Is a Story

This chapter discusses the treatment of disease, the body, or the patient. It first looks at identifying the best treatment and then moves on to the effects of patients on treatments. The concepts of placebo, treatment of the patient, and treatment in chronic illness are also discussed.

Treating the Disease, the Body, or the Patient

- Identifying the Best Treatment

- The Effects of Patients on Treatments

- The Placebo

- Treatment of This Patient

- Treatment in Chronic Illness

- Doctor, What is Going to Happen to Me?

This chapter discusses areas of medicine such as ethics to see how they would fare if medicine's primary focus were on something other than the disease itself.

It begins by examining the problems that would arise if the sick person became the central concern of medicine and physicians. The chapter then examines the search for a new basis for clinical medicine and provides a number of solutions.

This chapter discusses knowing and attempting to know a person over some time. It is believed that individuals are unknowable in their entirety due to the fact that people change constantly and that a person can only see one aspect of an individual at any moment.

The chapter discusses how to know people through their narratives and looks at personal logic, social constraints, and disinterest in the nature of the person.

This chapter discusses three kinds of information, namely empirical facts, value-laden terms, and aesthetics. It shows that this information about sick persons is necessary for the work of clinicians, and it also attempts to show that clinicians treat particular patients in particular circumstances at particular moments in time, thus requiring information that particularizes the individual and the moment.

This chapter discusses the experience of the clinician, beginning with the science and art of the practice of medicine. It then moves on to the importance of the clinician's experience, the relation of knowledge to experience, and why experience has a bad name.

The chapter then discusses the advantage of experience, the physician as the instrument, and how experience is able to mediate between science and art. It also looks at the experience of uncertainty.

This chapter discusses and examines the question: how does the mind act on the body? It presents a thesis that pertains to meanings and the things people do, the former being essential to the latter.

The chapter examines the concept of the mind while considering the concept of disease to be misleading. It discusses psychosomatic medicine, how the activities of thought influence the body, the flow of meaning, the coda, and the special case of preverbal children.

This chapter discusses dying. It presents two cases of women who have breast cancer, which demonstrate that there are meanings attached to the visible symbols of a disease or illness. Some of these meanings are related to the ideas of powerlessness.

This chapter discusses pain and suffering. It is concerned with symptoms and how the nature of the person modifies them. The chapter looks at the two steps of pain before looking at its progression to suffering and also looks at the failure to treat suffering, which is a phenomenon that cannot be separated from suffering.

BIOLOGY OF DISEASES

- Genes and gene products, molecular, cellular, and physiological structures and functions

- Biological factors linked to ethnicity, age, gender, pregnancy, and body weight.

- Endogenous biological factors or pathways involved in responses to infection or damage by external factors

- Metastases, degenerative processes, regeneration, and repair

- Complications, reoccurrence, and secondary conditions

- Bioinformatics and structural studies

- Development and characterization of models

- Environmental or external factors associated with the cause, risk, or development of disease, conditions, or ill health, including:

- Physical agents, occupational hazards, environmental surroundings, radiation, and pollution

Chemicals and nutrients infection by pathogens - bacteria, fungi, viruses, and other types of pathogens associated with social, psychological, and economic factors, including:

- Individual or group behaviors and lifestyle

- Cultural or religious beliefs or practices

- Ethnicity, age, and gender differences

- Socioeconomic factors

Proof that the causes of disease require more rigorous evidence. To identify novel factors associated with human disease, one may use a sequence-based where no etiology can be ascertained; the disorder is said to be idiopathic.

However, proof of causation in infectious diseases is limited to individual cases that provide experimental evidence of etiology.

Several lines of evidence together are required for causal inference for infectious cause disease fall into five groups: viruses, bacteria, fungi, protozoa, and helminths (worms). Sometimes, several symptoms always appear together, or more often than what could be expected, though it is known that one cannot cause the other. These situations are called syndromes.

Sometimes, there is no single cause of a disease; instead, there is a chain of causation from an initial trigger to the development of the clinical disease.

An example of all the above, which was recognized late, is that peptic ulcer disease may be induced by stress, requires the presence of acid secretion in the stomach, and has primary etiology in *Helicobacter pylori* infection. Many chronic diseases of unknown cause may be studied in this framework to explain multiple epidemiological associations.

Some diseases, such as diabetes or hepatitis, are syndromic allies defined by their signs and symptoms but include different conditions with different aetiologies. These are called heterogeneous conditions.

An **endotype** is a subtype of a condition that is defined by a distinct functional or path biological mechanism - One example is asthma, which is considered to be a syndrome consisting of a series of endotypes.

Another example could be AIDS, where an HIV infection can produce several clinical stages.

Classifications of diseases

Classifications of diseases become extremely important in the compilation of statistics on causes of illness (morbidity) and causes of death (mortality).

It is important to know what illnesses and diseases are prevalent in an area and how these prevalence rates vary over time.

With this knowledge, a search was instituted for possible causes of this increased prevalence.

The most widely used classifications of disease are (1) topographic, by bodily region or system; (2) anatomic, by organ or tissue; (3) physiological, by function or effect; (4) pathological, by the nature of the disease process, (5) etiologic (causal), (6) juristic, by the speed of advent of death, (7) epidemiological, and (8) statistical. Any single disease may fall within several of these classifications.

In the topographic classification, diseases are subdivided into such categories as gastrointestinal disease, vascular disease, abdominal disease, and chest disease.

In the anatomic classification, the disease is categorized by the specific organ or tissue affected; hence, heart disease, liver disease, and lung disease.

The physiological classification of disease is based on the underlying functional derangement produced by a specific disorder. Included in this classification are such designations as respiratory and metabolic disease

Metabolic diseases are those in which disturbances of the body's chemical processes are a basic feature. Diabetes and gout are examples.

The pathological classification of disease considers the nature of the disease process. Neoplastic and inflammatory diseases are examples.

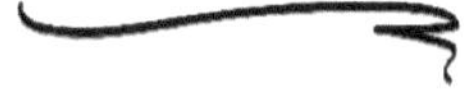

CONVENTIONAL VS. ALTERNATIVE MEDICINES

1) How does chronic disease alternative medicine differ from conventional allopathic treatment?

Conventional allopathic treatment is organ-specific; hence, there are various specialties medical practitioners like. Ophthalmologists, nephrologists, cardiologists...In modern medicine treatment, most disorders are traced to chemical imbalances and are treated with powerful chemicals (drugs).

Alternative medicine covers a broad range of healing philosophies, approaches, and therapies. It stimulates life energy and corrects the body's internal homeostasis. This can be applied to any disease. Very common alternative medicines are Homeopathy, Ayurveda, naturopathy, reiki, acupuncture, hypnotherapy, etc. Each system has its characteristics and benefits to give healing and cure so that a combined approach can give the best result as per one's expectations in chronic diseases.

2) For chronic diseases, does alternative medicine give good results or provide a total cure?

When illnesses are not infectious but due to body degeneration or dysfunction like heart disease, diabetes, arthritis, osteoporosis, etc., most conventional medicines don't correct the underlying pathology. And long-term uses of drugs slowly deteriorate the conditions.

Chronic diseases can be cured through a combined approach of various systems of medicine like Ayurveda, homeopathy, naturopathy, .etc. It can make organ dysfunctions normal and give permanent cures, and alternative medicine can avoid many surgeries.

3) How does alternative medicine treatment for chronic disease differ from conventional allopathic treatment?

In allopathic medicine, the result of the disease is targeted so relief is assured, but the disease process is not reversed. The original disease process remains as it is in the body. Alternative medicine tries to correct the root of the disease. And so makes it free.

The body has an inbuilt capacity to heal. Alternative medicine utilizes these bodies' healing power. If we know how to cooperate with the body's restorative powers, tremendous suffering could be avoided, but people don't know the right method. People often miss out on effective therapies and lack the information and support they need.

4) For chronic disease treatment, which has surety results?

The healing forces are present within the body. The body is constantly reacting between its internal environment and between its internal and external environment. It should be the physician's role to assist the body's natural state of homeostasis by cooperating with the body's efforts to heal so that the body gets cured of the disease and its root cause is removed. Alternative medicine puts the body in absolutely natural condition - physically and spiritually. Alternative medicine stimulates life energy within the body, and a complete cure for chronic diseases is possible.

5) How does alternative medicine differ from the present medical care system (Conventional medicine)?

Conventional medicine believes in specifically targeting the organ. Conventional medicine is organ-specific; hence, specialists and super specialists like ophthalmologists, cardiologists, nephrologists, and neurologists. Etc. Alternative medicine considers each person as one body. Conventional medicine understands organ and cellular chemical changes.

The philosophy behind alternative medicine is that nature includes all human bodies and has all the ingredients to treat any disharmony.

Alternative medicine utilizes life energy for cures, corrects imbalances in life, and strengthens this life energy, which is the ultimate goal of alternative medicine.

Alternative medicine believes in gentle, long-term support to enable the body's innate powers to heal, so there is a harmless approach. Conventional medicine believes in an aggressive approach so that the drugs can have toxic reactions.

In the modern medical care system, the focus is often on treating the disease and not the person. Alternative medicine goes into depth regarding diseases, and mental and physical matters are taken into consideration.

Investigation, procedures, surgery, chemotherapy, radiation, and powerful drugs can be avoided by alternative medicine. Even many major and minor surgeries can also be avoided.

For alternative medicine, pharmaceutical and other allied medical industrial complexes are no concern, so it is much more economical. Alternative medicine is devoid of a propaganda budget for hospitals and doctors, so again, it is much more economical.

Multinational business giants are connected with conventional medicine-making multispecialty hospitals and pharmaceutical companies. Manipulations at any level are possible. There are no such alternative medicines.

Hospital infections, surgery complications, and adverse drug reactions cause iatrogenic diseases and can cause death. In alternative medicines, there is no death due to their practice. It is harmless - Many alternative medicinal substances do not come within the preview of Regulatory Systems of /government. Conventional medicine is preferred in the treatment of trauma and emergencies, while alternative medicine excels in the treatment of chronic disease. The allopathic drug provides symptomatic relief, while the natural remedy is intended to remove the root cause of the disease. - We must have an eye to see it, see each system with respect, and not consider this as fake.

6) Which chronic diseases can be effectively treated by alternative medicine?

Some of the common diseases can be treated completely by alternative medicine, though any bodily disease can be treated by combined alternative medicine. For your further information, I am also giving you time to determine which total cure is possible. This is not only writing, but I can prove this in total curing number of times for many of my patients.

Cure in short time (3 to 4 months)	Flatulence –Dysentery – Constipation-Acidity
	Stress – Depression - Headache
	Throat - Allergy – Chronic Cold - Cough
	Pregnancy-Related Problems
	Old Age Problems - Premature Senility
	Acne – Boil -Abscess
	Skin-Itching - Urticaria
Cure in moderate time (6 to 9 months)	Liver Diseases -Gall Stone – Fissure –Piles- Ulcer
	Neuralgia –Insomnia - Twitching
	Heart Function - Hypertension
	Back Ache- Spondylitis –Gout -Joint Pain
	KIDNEY-Calculi

	Hair-Fall / Dandruff -Skin Warts
Cure in a long time (12 to 18 months)	Child Growth And Behavior Problems
	Vertigo
	Arthritis –Osteoarthritis - Spinal Affection
	Diabetes –Obesity -Eczema

7.) For chronic disease treatment, which different kinds of alternative medicines are available?

There are more than 400 alternative medicines all over the world, but the following have been very common in use: - (details of how it works and what strategies are beyond the inclusion of this write-up).

- Ayurveda

- Homeopathy

- Chiropractics

- Hypnotherapy

- Acupuncture

- Reiki

- Osteopathy

- Yoga

- Meditation

- Aromatherapy

8.) For chronic disease treatment, why do people not think of alternative medicines first? For chronic disease treatment, why are alternative medicines not so popular?

Whenever any bodily ailment is there, more commonly, people think of modern medical - allopathic - aspects only. Because we are filled with information on modern medicine only and hardly know alternative medicine. In all medical colleges, only modern medical science (allopathy) is taught. In modern medical sciences, alternative medicine is not taught in college. Also, in many countries, alternative medicine is not recognized. Also, guidance and treatment with alternative medicine are not available so easily. So, for their bodily ailments, very few people think of the line of alternative medicines. Few do not have any idea about the existence of alternative medicines!

It is embarked (detailed literature of diseases suffered are given for education) to believe that the system of modern medicine- allopathy is the only valid one and that all other natural medicines or alternative medicines are more or less just quackery.

Alternative medicine covers a broad range of healing philosophies, approaches, and therapies. The history of alternative medicine is long for many years and has sustained time's testing. So, it is easy to understand that a combined approach can give the best result as per one's expectations. It is very important to know the opinion of experts all over the world that allopathic medicine will not offer a complete cure for chronic diseases. In contrast, alternative medicine, as it stimulates life energy within the body, makes a complete cure for chronic diseases possible.

One of the reasons why alternative medicine is not more popular with the medical profession and the public is that it is too simple. The average mind is more impressed by the involved, mysterious, and complex management. But one thing is certain: those who one time take the help of alternative medicine will always employ alternative medicine systems only. Now, alternative medicine is not an "alternative" at all; rather, it is the basis of the healthcare system.

9.) What is the recent trend worldwide for chronic disease treatment with alternative medicines?

Patients in Western countries are becoming more receptive to trying alternative techniques, and Satisfaction expressed by many patients with alternative medicine is increasing. Some hospitals and doctors are supplementing their regular medical care with alternative techniques.

So, the inquiry was mounted because there is a widespread perception that CAM (complementary and alternative medicine) use is increasing, not only in the United Kingdom and the USA but across the developed world. Many of these "alternative" techniques come from all over the globe and have been around for thousands of years. The following govt sponsored organizations surveyed CAM (complementary and alternative medicine)

1) Research Council for Complementary Medicine, the School of Integrated Health at the University of Westminster. UK

2) National Center for Complementary and Alternative Medicine (NCCAM), a component of the National Institutes of Health, USA

3) www.parliament.uk > Publications and Records > Select Committees > Science and Technology

4) New York Online Access to Health.

5) Complementary and Alternative Medicine Website, New Zealand Guidelines Group

All the details cannot be included here, but all the authorities found a steep increase in the use of CAM.

The American Hospital Association reported that more than a quarter of the hospitals in a 2005 survey offered some alternative therapies like Homeopathy, Herbal support, biofeedback, or acupuncture. Its results suggest that there are approximately 50,000 CAM practitioners in the United Kingdom, that there are approximately 10,000 statutory registered health professionals who practice some form of CAM in the United Kingdom, and that up to 5 million patients have consulted a CAM practitioner in the last year. £450 million worth of out-of-pocket expenditure was used on six of the principal therapies (excluding aromatherapy and reflexology) during the preceding year.

10.) Chronic disease treatment with alternative medicines: How does it give the best results?

Chronic disease is a very tragic, emotionally damaging, and painful experience. Human beings are infused with a subtle form of energy. This vital energy or life force is known under different names in different cultures. It aims to integrate the body, mind, and spirit to prevent and treat disease. Vital energy is believed to flow throughout the human body, but it has not been measured by means of conventional instrumentation. Alternative medicines mobilize the body's vital force to orchestrate coordinated healing responses throughout the organism. The body translates the information on the vital force into local physical changes that lead to recovery from chronic diseases. This not only treats the main problem but can change a life, enthuse enjoyment in your life, and remove diseases from their root cause. While modern - allopathic medicine does not do so.

In allopathic management, underlying conditions often deteriorate despite the often brilliant diagnosis, medical management, or surgical correction. Most chronic illnesses cannot be cured completely. Frequently, the result is a lifetime of discomfort, doctor's visits, medical tests, medications, therapies, and sometimes surgeries. Some patients may become disabled or depressed due to enduring lengthy or recurring bouts of illness. Because of these factors, patients suffering from chronic disease disrupt other areas of their lives.

So, one must understand that chronic diseases can be cured through a combined approach of various systems of medicine.

11.) What can we expect from alternative medicines for chronic disease treatment? Whether this will work for me? What is the time limit?

Chronic disease often requires extensive care. No one can predict what the outcome of treatment is going to be for any chronic disease, and the final result is uncertain. Managing chronic diseases requires better practice systems, improved and extra doctors' skills, and more effective use of various alternative medicines. This is complex, and the management needs to be multi-faceted, multi-institutional, and sustainable. It should be clear in the first consultation how much time it will take, what the approach will be, and what the cost of treatment will be. Every patient should become healthier soon after the start of treatment, and it is this that gives the sign of how far the final result is. At the end of treatment, all patients must be satisfied with the good care, and they are definitely cured or better.

12.) I can still not decide to submit to you for treatment. How can I be sure? And how can I have an advantage in your treatment?

It is hard to find honest, expert advice that can truly solve life's biggest problems facing you. Many times, we want not only a Doctor but a guide/teacher/ friend who can understand the root cause of our problem and treat not only the problem but also teach us the way we should live - a person who can improve the quality of our life by applying easy and economical methods.

We constantly see in our family or our friends' circle that people suffer from chronic diseases. They go on taking medicines- spend lots and lots of money but never get healthy- on the contrary, they go on deteriorating. Mostly, they have no idea how to get well. Most simply, they take it for granted that they will be well with medicines or surgeries. Unfortunately, this is not always the case. Few others rush into treatment without proper planning. The overall impact of chronic diseases on individuals differs greatly and is influenced by many factors, such as cultural background and individual life. Etc. This can be discussed only in terms of psychological factors. Very meticulous people - make all decisions perfectly and fail to plan for their treatment. Tremendous suffering could be avoided, but people don't know the right method. People often miss out on effective therapies and lack the information and support they need.

We are currently limited by a system that is built around treating acute episodes and responding to emergencies, not on effective management and cure of chronic medical conditions. It is embarked (detailed literature of diseases suffered are given for education) to believe that the system of modern medicine- allopathy is the only valid one and that all other natural medicines or patients are more or less just quackery.

When you are so fine and judgmental, you will certainly have the insight to know what truth is and what is false. Leave this decision to your inner jury to judge and to decide and follow what your inner jury has ordered. You have the right to ask as many questions as you can. It is a law of the universe that you have to be true to all human beings. If you do not remain, the universe will take very drastic actions, which will be very hard to bear. Be a fearing person and believe in giving the best to humanity.

Doctors are considered God and should offer good scope for satisfactory solutions to give the final cure to any chronic disease at an almost very low cost and in less time.

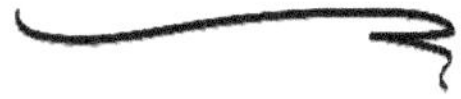

CHRONIC DISEASES
UNDERSTANDING

Chronic Diseases - Understanding

What is a chronic disease? And know-how of chronic disease.

A chronic disease lasts for three months or more. Chronic diseases generally cannot be prevented by vaccines or cured by allopathic medication, nor do they just disappear. Chronic diseases tend to become more common with age. Now, with the increased aged population, there is an increased prevalence of chronic diseases. Eighty-eight percent of Americans over 65 years of age have at least one chronic health condition.

The human body sends out a flare when something's awry. -- You should keep in mind unexplained weight loss and loss of appetite, Slurred speech, paraesthesia, weakness, tingling, burning pains, numbness, confusion, sudden agonizing headache, irregular bleeding from any organ

Modern medicine is organ-specific, hence various specialties like... ophthalmologists, cardiologists, nephrologists, neurologists... etc. Each specialist treats their disease by aggressive intervention, and the focus is often on treating the disease and not the person. In modern medicine treatment, most disorders are traced to chemical imbalances and are treated with powerful chemicals (drugs).

Chronic diseases have a prolonged course of illness. Chronic diseases contribute much to illness, disability-morbidity, and mortality. When illnesses are not infectious but due to body degeneration like heart disease, diabetes, arthritis, osteoporosis, etc, most drugs don't correct the pathology. Long-term use of drugs never gets people quite better and slowly deteriorates due to side effects of the drugs, development of poor immune function, and advancing age problems. As time goes by, more problems are "discovered"-more organs are involved, so more drugs are prescribed. At some point, the conditions can become so severe that they just do nothing and wait for the end.

This is where we must have to adjust our thinking toward consideration of the other system of medicine. We need to know how to cooperate with the body's restorative powers. Tremendous suffering could be avoided, but people don't know the right method. People often miss out on effective therapies and lack the information and support they need.

Chronic diseases can be cured through a combined approach of various systems of medicine like Ayurvedic, homeopathy, naturopathy ...etc. One will be amazed to see the result after employing various systems of medicine.

We are currently limited by a system that is built around treating acute episodes and responding to emergencies, not on effective management and cure of chronic medical conditions. It is embarked (detailed literature of diseases suffered are given for education) to believe that the system of modern medicine- allopathy is the only valid one and that all other natural medicines or patients are more or less just quackery.

Hearing the name of diseases, we immediately think of the line of pathophysiology. Immediately, we are supplied by the hospital with all the details of the disease we are suffering from. We get knowledge - what is disease? Where is the fault? We go on taking medicine or submit for surgery, but we do not ask the question of whether this medicine or surgical procedure will have the final cure. We hardly think or believe, or we do not have any idea that alternative medicine can correct such surgical pathology. The truth is that alternative medicine can prevent many surgeries. Hardly people have thought of adopting alternative medicine. Alternative medicine covers a broad range of healing philosophies, approaches, and therapies. The history of alternatives is long, many, many years, and it has sustained time testing. So, it is easy to understand that a combined approach can give the best result as per one's expectations.

God has created such a system that the healing forces are present within the body. The body is constantly reacting between its internal and external environment. The physician's role should be to assist the body's natural state of homeostasis by cooperating with the body's efforts to heal so that the body gets cured of the disease and its root cause is removed. Alternative medicine puts the body in absolutely natural condition – physically and spiritually. It is very important to know the opinion of experts all over the world that allopathic medicine will not offer a complete cure for chronic diseases. In contrast, alternative medicine, as it stimulates life energy within the body, makes a complete cure for chronic diseases possible.

Now, alternative medicine is not an "alternative" at all; rather, it is the basis of the healthcare system.

More understanding of chronic disease.

Many National bodies suggest such changes, but all of these changes are generalized and could take years to produce gains in the population's health. We, ourselves, must alter processes and priorities for ourselves.

Sustained improvements in managing chronic diseases require better practice systems, improvement in doctors' skills, and more effective use of various alternative medicines.

Patients should be treated as per their constitution and requirements, which vary from individual to individual. Just after the start of the treatment with alternative medicines, all patients are satisfied, and there is definite improvement.

Alternative medicine offers positive health changes to a substantial proportion of a large cohort of patients with a wide range of chronic diseases. One of the reasons why alternative medicine is not more popular with the medical profession and the public is that it is too simple. The average mind is more impressed by the involved, mysterious, and complex management. But one thing is certain: those who one time take the help of alternative medicine will always employ alternative medicine systems only.

Carry home message is do not suffer from chronic diseases for yourself or in your family and get a total cure to remove the root cause of disease.

Alternative medicine covers a broad range of healing philosophies, approaches, and therapies. Each system has its characteristics and benefits that help heal and cure many ailments for human beings. Each system of alternate medicine claims a high cure in its way, so it is easy to understand that a combined approach can give the best result as per one's expectations.

So why not take advantage of the various systems? The advantages of various systems of medicine should be combined to offer the best approach for management. This may give results faster, with less suffering, and in an economical way.

Chronic diseases are a very tragic, emotionally damaging, and painful experience. **Each patient requires sympathy towards their problem, and all their quarries should be solved with utmost satisfaction.** Every individual and patient handles the emotions of chronic disease treatment differently. An individualized approach is of utmost importance. A sympathetic, human, and heartfelt approach is a must. It is helpful when beginning chronic disease treatment to develop a perfect plan so that patients can have an idea of how long to pursue a particular treatment...

In Far East countries like Japan – Taiwan –Korea – and china - people live for long years and are healthy. WHY? They first depend on their herbal medicine and believe in nature. Healing forces are present within the body; you have to cooperate with the body's restorative powers.

We constantly see in our family or our friends' circle that people suffer from chronic diseases. They go on taking medicines- spend lots and lots of money but never get healthy.

In today's world of commercialism, people often miss out on effective therapies and lack the information and support they need.

When illnesses are due to body degeneration, like heart disease, diabetes, arthritis, osteoporosis, etc., most drugs don't correct the underlying pathology. Long-term use of drugs never gets people better but slowly deteriorates due to side effects of the drugs, development of poor immune function, and advancing age problems. As time goes by, more problems are "discovered"- more organs are involved, so more drugs are prescribed - and this circle goes on. At some point, the conditions can become so severe that they just do nothing and wait for the end.

Do not suffer from chronic diseases for yourself or your family, and get the total cure to remove the root cause of the disease. Tremendous suffering could be avoided, but people don't know the right method.

The body has all the ingredients to make healing on its own, but we need to know how to cooperate with the body's restorative powers.

Chronic diseases can be cured through a combined approach of various systems of medicine like Ayurvedic, homeopathy, naturopathy ...etc. One will be amazed to see the result after employing various systems of medicine. This gives results faster, with less suffering, and in an economical way. A combined approach of various alternative medicines can cover a broad range of healing philosophies, approaches, and therapies that will correct body degeneration and give definite and good results.

The great thing about these ancient remedies is that they usually do not have the health risks that some modern techniques and medications have today. All you need is to make a perfect and intelligent decision.

In medical colleges, only modern medical science (allopathy) is taught. In these modern medical colleges, alternative medicine is not taught. Also, in some countries, not all alternative medicines are recognized. Also, guidance and treatment with alternative medicine are not available so easily. So, for their bodily ailments, very few people think of the line of alternative medicines. Few do not have any idea about the existence of alternative medicines!

Alternative medicine stimulates life energy within the body; a complete cure from chronic diseases is possible. Alternative medicine can also correct surgical pathology so that surgeries can be avoided. This stimulates healing on the physical, emotional, and spiritual levels to restore vitality and creative engagement in life.

Now, alternative medicine is not an "alternative" at all; rather, it is the basis of the healthcare system.

A body constitution and body requirement varies from individual to individual. Every individual and patient handles the changes of chronic diseases differently. An individualized approach is of utmost importance. **Healing forces are present within the body, and the physician's role should be to assist the body's natural state of homeostasis by cooperating with bodies efforts to heal it.**

Sustained improvements in managing chronic diseases require better practice systems, very high doctors' skills, and more effective use of various alternative medicines.

Trust and the doctor-patient relationship are of utmost importance. Ultimately, whatever doctors do is for the benefit of patients only. The doctor is not GOD. Doctors can only try to give the maximum possible results.

Alternative Medicine Gives Amazing Cure for Chronic Diseases.

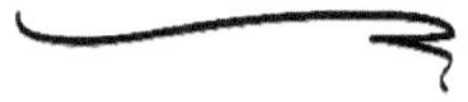

ALLOPATHIC MEDICINES

Allopathic medicine is another term for conventional or modern Western medicine. It is an evidence-based system in which doctors and other healthcare professionals treat symptoms using conventional medications.

The terms "allopathic medicine" and "allopathy" are derived from the Greek prefix ἄλλος (állos), meaning "other," "different," and the suffix πάθος (páthos), meaning "suffering."

Hahnemann and other early homeopaths used the term allopath to highlight the difference they perceived between homeopathy and the "conventional." With the term allopathy (meaning "other than the disease"), Hahnemann intended to point out how physicians employed therapeutic approaches[1]

Hahnemann used "allopathy" to refer to what he saw as a system of medicine that combats disease by using remedies that produce effects in a healthy subject. The distinction comes from the use in homeopathy of substances that are meant to cause similar effects as the symptoms of a disease to treat patients (*homeo* - meaning "similar").

As used by homeopaths, the term *allopathy* has always referred to the principle of treating disease by administering substances that produce other symptoms. For example, part of an allopathic treatment for fever may include the use of a drug that reduces the fever while also including a drug (such as an antibiotic) that attacks the cause of the fever (such as a bacterial infection). A homeopathic treatment for fever, by contrast, uses a diluted dosage of a substance that, in an undiluted form, would induce fever in a healthy person. These preparations are typically diluted so heavily that they no longer contain any actual molecules of the original substance. Hahnemann used this term to distinguish medicine as practiced in his time from his use of infinitesimally small doses of substances to treat the spiritual causes of illness.

World Health Organization (WHO) in 2001 defined "allopathic medicine" as "the broad category of medical practice that is sometimes called Western medicine, biomedicine, evidence-based medicine, or modern medicine."

Homeopathy	Medicine
"A system of therapeutics founded by Samuel Hahnemann (1755-1843), based on the Law of Similars where "like cures like." Diseases are treated by highly diluted substances that cause, in healthy persons, symptoms like those of the disease to be treated."	"The art and science of studying, performing research on, preventing, diagnosing, and treating disease, as well as the maintenance of health"

"A system of complementary medicine in which ailments are treated by minute doses of natural substances that in larger amounts would produce symptoms of the ailment"	"The science or practice of the diagnosis, treatment, and prevention of disease.
"A system of medical practice that aims to combat disease by use of remedies (as drugs or surgery) producing effects different from or incompatible with those produced by the disease being treated"	"The science and art dealing with the maintenance of health and the prevention, alleviation, or cure of disease"

Allopathic medicine is another term for conventional Western medicine. Allopathy uses mainstream medical practices like diagnostic blood work, prescription drugs, and surgery.[1]

An allopathic doctor is typically an MD, while osteopaths (DO), chiropractors (DC), and Asian medical doctors (OMD) usually fall under the complementary medicine umbrella.

Modern medicine grew largely from the discoveries made since the scientific revolution and the ongoing linkage of medical knowledge to rigorous research methods. The coupling of expert knowledge to compassionate delivery of care—modern medicine—is often held out as one of the most tangible examples of human progress. It produced a dynamic, self-correcting system that evolves and makes use of discoveries to deliver the best patient care possible.

But not everybody came along for the ride. The progress of scientific medicine continues in stark contrast with other sectarian, cultural, and overtly religious belief systems related to human health. These remained static, and there needs to be more to distinguish between belief systems like naturopathy, homeopathy, chiropractic, traditional Chinese medicine, and so on today from the practices as they were originally constituted.

In the early 1800s, a schism developed between medical practitioners who espoused the beliefs of Hahnemann, the inventor of homeopathy (where infinitely dilute preparations of toxic substances are purported to cure illness), and those who felt such ideas were inadequate.

Hahnemann himself coined the term allopath. The term was intended to indicate, in a derogatory way, that conventional practitioners of the early 19th century only treated disease by opposing symptoms and offered nothing in terms of preventing illness or addressing the root causes of disease.

The term allopath was rejected by mainstream medicine but has continued to be used by homeopaths and other unconventional practitioners when referring to medical doctors. While physicians of the early 1800s had much less to offer patients than they do today, a knowledge of anatomy, the natural history of many diseases, and the early appreciation of the microbial causes of infectious diseases had begun to allow physicians to do far more.

Indeed, as time went on, conventional medicine began to develop and deploy discoveries such as vaccines, insulin, new medicines and surgeries, cancer therapies, and public health campaigns that not only treated symptoms but effectively eliminated a large number of diseases and prevented many others.

It is all the more ironic, then, that the term allopath has become more commonly and effectively leveled by adherents of complementary/alternative/integrative therapies in the medical profession. Perhaps unknowingly, some physicians apply the term to their trade, not understanding that the term connotes a practitioner very different from themselves.

The word is derived from the Greek allos (against) and pathos (suffering) and really denotes a process of diminishing symptoms. Notably, modern medicine has done more to understand, treat, cure, and prevent disease than any other entity in the history of humankind.

More interestingly, depicting scientific medicine as allopathic medicine is often used as a device to define debate at an administrative level when unconventional practitioners wish to position themselves as equal partners on the healthcare playing field.

The BCMA has heard this from the mouths of government officials in the discussions around the scope of practice, and it appears with some regularity in the submissions of unconventional practitioners to health ministries when the extra status is being sought.

When advocating for scarce government health dollars, it sounds so much better to offer naive administrators a choice between naturopathic, homeopathic, allopathic, Native healing, and Eastern medicine than it does to tell the truth: that you can choose between medicine that's consistent with the best information available, or things that aren't.—Lloyd Oppel, MD Chair, Allied Health and Alternative Therapies Committee.

What Is an Allopathic Doctor?

- What Does an Allopathic Doctor Do?

- Education and Training

- Reasons to See an Allopathic Doctor

Maybe an allopathic doctor has helped you or treated you at some point during your lifetime. These medical professionals treat conditions, symptoms, or diseases using a range of drugs, surgery, or therapies.

Simply put, an allopathic doctor practices modern medicine. Other terms for allopathic medicine include Western, orthodox, mainstream, or conventional medicine.

"Allo," which comes from the Greek word for "opposite," means to treat the symptom with its opposite. Allopathic doctors may specialize in a number of areas of clinical practice and have the title of medical doctor or MD.

What Does an Allopathic Doctor Do?

An allopathic doctor uses allopathic treatments to help people with a variety of conditions or diseases.

They may choose to focus on research or teaching throughout their career, in addition to choosing a field in which to specialize. They can be found in private practice, hospitals, medical centers, or clinics.

Medical doctors practice allopathic medicine rather than osteopathic medicine. More than 90% of doctors currently practicing in the United States have the title MD.

The other 10% are doctors of osteopathic medicine or osteopaths. They're similar to allopathic doctors in that they use a variety of modern medicine, technology, and drugs to treat people. However, they also incorporate holistic care and philosophy into their practice.

An allopathic doctor is certified to diagnose and treat illnesses in addition to performing surgery and prescribing medications. An allopathic doctor can get licensed to perform their duties in any of the 50 states of the United States.

Education and Training

All doctors who practice allopathy follow a similar path. First, they complete an undergraduate degree in a related field. Next, the candidate receives a satisfactory score on the Medical

College Admission Test (MCAT) and completes four years of medical school. After medical school, an allopathic doctor completes a residency program to get hands-on training alongside medical professionals. Depending on the specialty, a residency program can last from 3 to 7 years.

Some specialties in allopathy include:

- Cardiovascular medicine

- Neurology

- Oncology

- Pediatrics

- Surgery

- Family medicine

- Dermatology

- Orthopedics

- Internal medicine

The American Board of Medical Specialties recognizes 24 board-certified areas of specialties in allopathy. Within these specialties are many other subspecialties that an allopathic doctor may choose to focus on.

Reasons to See an Allopathic Doctor

You may visit an allopathic doctor for a number of reasons. You might go when you have symptoms that interfere with your daily life or well-being.

You should also seek out allopathic care if you have any of the following ongoing symptoms. While many are common in the short term, these symptoms may be signs of a larger problem if they don't go away.

- **Digestive problems like:**

    o   Constant heartburn

    o   Trouble swallowing

    o   Severe belly pain

    o   Ongoing constipation

    o   Diarrhea that lasts more than three days

    o   Blood in your poop

    o   Poop that's black and tar-like

    o   Back pain that's:

    o   Constant and spreads down your legs

    o   Accompanied by sweating, fever, swelling, or redness on your back

- **Period problems such as:**

    o   Severe cramps

    o   Irregular cycles

    o   Bleeding between cycles

    o   No cycle for more than three months

These are a few examples of when it might be time to get allopathic care. An allopathic doctor is committed to helping people and improving their health. They're there to listen, provide care, and help you improve your overall well-being.

What Is Allopathic Medicine?

Allopathic medicine refers to the practice of conventional Western medicine.[2] The term allopathic medicine is most often used to contrast conventional medicine with complementary medicine.

Integrative medicine is the term that is being increasingly used to refer to the practice of combining the best of complementary medicine with the best of conventional medicine to manage and reduce the risk of disease.

Allopathic medicine examples include:

- Antibiotics

- Blood work and laboratory testing

- Chemotherapy

- Hormone replacement therapy

- Insulin

- like Paracetamol (acetaminophen) and naproxen

- Primary care medicine

- Specialists in cardiology, endocrinology, oncology, and rheumatology

- Surgery

- Vaccines

- Ultrasounds

- X-rays

History of Allopathy

The term allopathic medicine was coined in the 1800s to differentiate two types of medicine.[4] Homeopathy was on one side, based on the theory that "like cures like."[5] The thought with homeopathy is that very small doses of a substance that causes the symptoms of a disease could be used to alleviate that disease.

In contrast, allopathic medicine was defined as the practice of using opposites: using treatments that have the opposite effects of the symptoms of a condition.

At the time, the term allopathic medicine was often used in a derogatory sense. It referred to radical treatments such as bleeding people to relieve fever. Over the years, this meaning has changed, and now the term encompasses most of the modern medicine in developed countries.

Current Allopathic Practices

Today, allopathic medicine is mainstream medicine. The term is no longer derogatory and instead describes current Western medicine. Most physicians are considered allopathic providers.

Medical insurance covers most types of allopathic care, whereas complementary medicine is often an out-of-pocket cost.

Examples of allopathic medicine include everything from primary care physicians to specialists and surgeons.

Other terms used interchangeably with allopathic medicine include:

- Conventional medicine

- Traditional Western medicine

- Orthodox medicine

- Mainstream medicine

- Biomedicine

- Evidence-based medicine

These allopathic monikers are usually contrasted with complementary practices, such as:

- Ayurveda

- Traditional Chinese Medicine

- Folk medicine

- Homeopathy

- Natural medicine or naturopathy

- Bioregulatory medicine

- Phototherapy

What Is Osteopathic Medicine?

Allopathic vs. Alternative Medicine

In the past, allopathic practitioners tended to look down on alternative medicine practitioners and vice versa. However, that is changing as more physicians find alternative practices that may be beneficial. This is particularly the case when a patient suffers from a chronic medical condition that lacks a "quick fix" with a pill or procedure.

Likewise, many alternative practitioners realize that allopathic medicine clearly has a role.[6] For example, if your appendix is inflamed and getting ready to burst, a holistic doctor would send you to a surgeon, which is an allopathic practitioner. Research shows both sides of medicine can be helpful, depending on the diagnosis.[7] A 2017 study found allopathic providers tend to care for people with concrete conditions like high blood pressure, heart disease, diabetes, and cancer. Alternative practitioners, on the other hand, tend to treat symptoms such as pain, congestion, and constipation.[7]

Today, allopathic and alternative medicine are being combined as a way to both treat conditions and relieve symptoms. This is known as integrative medicine.

What Is Integrative Medicine?

Integrative medicine practices aim to provide the best of both worlds. Conventional medicine is the primary treatment technique, and alternative therapies complement patient care.

Integrative care is commonly seen in many cancer centers. Allopathic medicine treatments like surgery, chemotherapy, and radiation are used to treat cancer. Alternative methods like acupuncture, meditation, and massage are used to treat the side effects of cancer treatments.[8]

Examples of alternative methods often used along with allopathic medicine include:

- Acupuncture

- Art therapy

- Massage therapy

- Meditation

- Music therapy

- Pet therapy

- Qigong

- Reiki

- Yoga

'It is modern medicine, not allopathy.'

Allopathy was the term coined by Samuel Hahnemann to denote a system of medicine that is opposed to homeopathy, which he founded.

The doctors on the dais pointed out that the term allopathy was outdated indeed. They said modern medicine was an evidence-based system that should be referred to as it is. The session was meant to shed light on the purported unscientific nature of alternative medical practices such as Ayurveda, Siddha, Unani, and Homeopathy. Questions were chosen from select participants.

DEFINITION OF ALLOPATHIC MEDICINE

The doctors on the dais pointed out that the term allopathy was outdated indeed. They said modern medicine was an evidence-based system that should be referred to as it is. The session was meant to shed light on the purported unscientific nature of alternative medical practices such as Ayurveda, Siddha, Unani, and Homeopathy. Questions were chosen from select participants.

ALLOPATHIC MEDICINES

Advantages and Disadvantages

- It focuses on the part, not complete health.

- Allopathic medicines may destroy good bacteria.

- Drugs don't cure; they suppress.

- Invasive procedures may be dangerous.

- Missing out on the whole picture.

- Allopathy doesn't assess the pros and cons.

- Allopathic medicine relies on Source clinical examinations and screening to confirm a diagnosis, focusing on a person's symptoms and signs before treatment.

- Allopathic medicine treatment modalities include Trusted Source pharmacological drugs, surgery, and radiation therapies.

- A patient is never considered as a person but as an assembly(assortment) of various organs.

- Every drug contains chemicals that are harmful to health, especially if used over a long period.

- No cure for any disease.

- Since allopathy can't cure any chronic diseases, they increasingly depend on surgery to prevent the recurrence of symptoms. In the process, they deprive the body of its original anatomy, which is necessary for its sustenance.

- Treatments are mainly aimed at suppressing diseases to bring quick relief to the patients. Damage caused to the people by such activities is ignored.

- The action of drugs is only at the tissue level. Hence, people with multiple diseases require multiple drugs.

- The human body is considered a machine. Specialists for each organ ignore the vital energy that synchronizes and optimizes the activities of different organs and systems. Hence, organ transplantation, fitting artificial parts, and replacement therapy have become common practice.

- Treatment aims to maintain biochemical and physiological values. Hence, frequent checking and other biochemical values are considered necessary for therapy.

- Most of the treatments are interventional; hence, complications (even life-threatening) are common.

- Since interventional treatments demand a lot of disposable materials and sophisticated equipment, the procedures could be more affordable.

- Since drugs are mostly strong chemicals, adverse reactions are possible

- Almost all drugs have serious side effects, which may surpass the disease proper, resulting in organ failure.

- They try to overcome the serious flaws in the treatment methods by including scientific gadgets and innovations to impress upon the patients.

- Allopathy is no longer a treatment method. But it's part of the healthcare industry aimed at profiteering, thereby losing any sanctity of service to humanity. People suffering are seen as opportunities for profiteering. Healthcare professionals are trained to be part of this system of helping each other to mint money.

- Allopathy treatment is more or less mechanical, and it has become the culture to disregard the patient as an individual. The doctor-patient relationship is almost non-existent.

- Flaws in treatment methodology are compensated by gimmicks like calling themselves 'modern medicine, ' scientific medicine, evidence-based medicine, etc., and ridiculing other systems of treatment as pseudoscience to enjoy monopoly in the future.

- Most of the healthcare professionals involved in allopathy are arrogant, contemptuous, and greedy. They have no time to listen to patients or too busy to say kind words to them.

- Allopathy treatment is simply unaffordable to the commoner or consciously made so to help health insurance companies.

There are many advantages of allopathic medicine; for example, Doctors have access to the latest technology to diagnose and treat illnesses and injuries. Allopathic doctors are highly skilled physicians who can treat illnesses and injuries and perform tests to help improve the quality of life of their patients.

Allopathy is known for its quick and targeted relief of symptoms, making it suitable for acute conditions or emergencies.

Why choose allopathic medicine?

The main benefit of allopathic medicine is its evidence-based system. This means each diagnostic tool and treatment regimen is the product of robust scientific research. Other benefits of allopathic care include receiving treatment from highly qualified and licensed professionals.

Allopathy focuses on treating a particular organ or area affected by an illness or condition. However, this approach risks side effects and the possibility of infection spreading to nearby areas. In contrast, homeopathy is generally considered safe since it does not have any adverse effects on other parts of the body.

ALLOPATHIC MEDICINES

Allopathic medicine is another term for conventional or modern Western medicine. It is an evidence-based system in which doctors and other healthcare professionals treat symptoms using conventional medications.

It was based on the belief that disease is caused by an imbalance of the four " (blood, phlegm, yellow bile, and black bile) and sought to treat disease symptoms by correcting that imbalance, using "harsh and abusive" methods to induce symptoms seen as opposite to those of diseases rather than treating their underlying causes: the disease was caused by an excess of one humor and thus would be treated with its "opposite."

The terms "allopathic medicine" and "allopathy" are derived from the Greek prefix ἄλλος (állos), meaning "other," "different," and the suffix πάθος (páthos), meaning "suffering."

Hahnemann and other early homeopaths used the term allopath to highlight the difference they perceived between homeopathy and the "conventional" heroic medicine of their time. With the term allopathy (meaning "other than the disease"), Hahnemann intended to point out how physicians with conventional training employed therapeutic approaches that, in his view, merely treated symptoms and failed to address the disharmony produced by an underlying disease.[clarification needed] Homeopaths saw such symptomatic treatments as "opposites treating opposites" and believed these methods were harmful to patients.

Hahnemann used "allopathy" to refer to what he saw as a system of medicine that combats disease by using remedies that produce effects in a healthy subject that are different (hence the Greek root allo- "different") from the effects produced by the disease to be treated.

The distinction comes from the use in homeopathy of substances that are meant to cause similar effects as the symptoms of a disease to treat patients (homeo - meaning "similar").

Within homeopathic practice, the term "allopathy" has consistently denoted the approach of treating illnesses by administering substances that provoke symptoms different from those of the disease when given to a healthy individual.

For instance, an allopathic remedy for fever might involve the use of a medication to reduce the fever alongside another drug, such as an antibiotic, to combat the underlying cause, such as a bacterial infection.

In contrast, a homeopathic approach to fever entails administering a highly diluted dosage of a substance that, in its pure form, would induce fever in a healthy person. These preparations are typically diluted to the extent that they no longer contain detectable molecules of the original substance. Hahnemann employed this term to distinguish conventional medicine of his era from his method of using infinitesimal doses of substances, or even none at all, to address the spiritual roots of illness.

Current usage

A study released by the World Health Organization (WHO) in 2001 defined "allopathic medicine" as "the broad category of medical practice that is sometimes called Western medicine, biomedicine, evidence-based medicine, or modern medicine.

Homeopathy	Medicine
"A system of therapeutics founded by Samuel Hahnemann (1755-1843), based on the Law of Similars where "like cures like." Diseases are treated by highly diluted substances that cause, in healthy persons, symptoms like those of the disease to be treated."	"The art and science of studying, performing research on, preventing, diagnosing, and treating disease, as well as the maintenance of health"
"A system of complementary medicine in which ailments are treated by minute doses of natural substances that in larger amounts would produce symptoms of the ailment"	"The science or practice of the diagnosis, treatment, and prevention of disease (in technical use often taken to exclude surgery."

Homeopathy	Medicine
"A system of medical practice that aims to combat disease by use of remedies (as drugs or surgery) producing effects different from or incompatible with those produced by the disease being treated"	"The science and art dealing with the maintenance of health and the prevention, alleviation, or cure of disease"

Allopathic medicine is another term for conventional Western medicine. In contrast to complementary medicine (sometimes known as alternative medicine), allopathy uses mainstream medical practices like diagnostic blood work, prescription drugs, and surgery.[1]

It produced a dynamic, self-correcting system that evolves and makes use of discoveries to deliver the best patient care possible.

While physicians of the early 1800s had much less to offer patients than they do today, a knowledge of anatomy, the natural history of many diseases, and the early appreciation of the microbial causes of infectious diseases had begun to allow physicians to do far more than was captured by the derogatory term.

Indeed, as time went on, conventional medicine began to develop and deploy discoveries such as vaccines, insulin, new medicines and surgeries, cancer therapies, and public health campaigns that not only treated symptoms but effectively eliminated a large number of diseases and prevented many others.

These medical professionals treat conditions, symptoms, or diseases using a range of drugs, surgery, or therapies.

Simply put, an allopathic doctor practices modern medicine. Other terms for allopathic medicine include Western, orthodox, mainstream, or conventional medicine.

Other terms used interchangeably with allopathic medicine include:

- Conventional medicine

- Traditional Western medicine

- Orthodox medicine

- Mainstream medicine

- Biomedicine

- Evidence-based medicine (Alternative medicine modalities can also be evidence-based if significant research has shown it works.)

These allopathic monikers are usually contrasted with complementary practices, such as:

- Ayurveda

- Traditional Chinese Medicine

- Folk medicine

- Homeopathy

- Natural medicine or naturopathy

- Bioregulatory medicine

- Phytotherapy

What Is Integrative Medicine?

Integrative medicine practices aim to provide the best of both worlds. Conventional medicine is the primary treatment technique, and alternative therapies complement patient care.

Integrative care is commonly seen in many cancer centers. Allopathic medicine treatments like surgery, chemotherapy, and radiation are used to treat cancer. Alternative methods like acupuncture, meditation, and massage are used to treat the side effects of cancer treatments.[8]

Examples of alternative methods often used along with allopathic medicine include

- Acupuncture

- Art therapy

- Massage therapy

- Meditation

- Music therapy

- Pet therapy

- Qigong

- Reiki

- Yoga

- The doctors on the dais pointed out that the term allopathy was outdated indeed. They said modern medicine was an evidence-based system that should be referred to as it is. The session was meant to shed light on the purported unscientific nature of alternative medical practices such as Ayurveda, Siddha, Unani, and Homeopathy. Questions were chosen from select participants.

- The doctors on the dais pointed out that the term allopathy was outdated indeed. They said modern medicine was an evidence-based system that should be referred to as it is. The session was meant to shed light on the purported unscientific nature of alternative medical practices such as Ayurveda, Siddha, Unani, and Homeopathy. Questions were chosen from select participants.

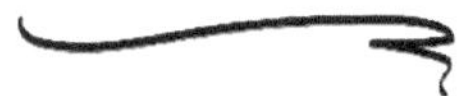

AYURVEDIC SYSTEM

Ayurveda treatment starts with an internal purification process, followed by a special diet, herbal remedies, massage therapy, yoga, and meditation.

Ayurveda: Does It Really Work?

Ayurveda (a Sanskrit word that means "science of life" or "knowledge of life") is one of the world's oldest whole-body healing systems. It was developed more than 5,000 years ago in India.

Ayurveda is based on the belief that health and wellness depend on a delicate balance between the mind, body, spirit, and environment. The main goal of Ayurvedic medicine is to promote good health and prevent, not fight, disease. However, treatments may be geared toward specific health problems.

Ayurveda is one of the oldest holistic healing systems in the world. It suggests that your health is based on the balance between your mind, body, spirit, and environment. (Photo Credit: iStock/Getty Images)

Ayurveda and Your Life Energy

Ayurveda is based on the theory that everything in the universe – dead or alive – is connected- interlinked. If your mind, body, and spirit are in harmony with the universe, you have good health. When something disrupts this balance, you get sick. Among the things that can upset this balance are genetic or congenital disabilities, injuries, climate and seasonal change, age, and emotions.

Those who practice Ayurveda believe every person is made of five basic elements found in the universe: space, air, fire, water, and earth.

These combine in the human body to form three life forces, or energies, called doshas. They control how your body works. They are Vata dosha (space and air), pitta dosha (fire and water), and Kapha dosha (water and earth).

Everyone inherits a unique mix of the three doshas, but one is usually stronger than the others. Each one controls a different body function. It's believed that the balance of your doshas is linked to your chances of getting sick and the health issues you develop.

The Three Doshas in Ayurveda

Vata dosha

Those who practice Ayurveda believe this is the most powerful of all three doshas. It controls very basic body functions, like how cells divide. It also controls your mind, breathing, blood flow, heart function, and the ability to get rid of waste through your intestines. Things that can disrupt it include eating again too soon after a meal, fear, grief, and staying up too late.

If Vata is your dominant dosha, you may be smart, creative, and vibrant, and your moods change quickly. Physically, you may be thin, lose weight easily, and are usually cold.

When you are out of balance, you can get overstimulated, have anxiety and phobias, and be forgetful. You can also be more likely to have conditions like asthma, heart disease, skin problems, and rheumatoid arthritis.

In Ayurveda, like increases like. For this dosha (space and air), you can balance out too much vata by doing grounding things like meditation, massage, keeping a regular sleep and wake schedule, and eating warm, mild foods.

Pitta dosha

This energy controls your digestion, metabolism (how well you break down foods), and certain hormones that are linked to your appetite. Things that can disrupt pitta are eating sour or spicy foods, spending too much time in the sun, and missing meals.

If you are pitta dominant, then you may be goal-oriented, competitive, confident, and a natural leader. Physically, you may have a medium-sized, muscular build and tend to be hot most of the time.

When out of balance, you can be too competitive, cranky, quick to anger, and impulsive. If pitta is your main dosha, you're thought to be more likely to have conditions like Crohn's disease, heart disease, high blood pressure, indigestion, and fever.

To bring pitta (fire and water) back into balance, you can focus on things that are cooling and light, like salads and cucumbers, and practice moderation and slow or restorative yoga.

Kapha dosha

Kapha dosha is thought to control muscle growth, body strength and stability, weight, and your immune system. Things that can disrupt kapha include daytime naps, eating too many sweet foods, and eating or drinking things that contain too much salt or water.

If Kapha is your main dosha, you may like routine, stick to expectations, and be accepting, calm, and patient. Physically, you are more likely to have a broad frame and easily gain weight.

When out of balance, you can easily get fatigued, avoid taking on new projects, and be possessive, stubborn, and depressed. If you are kapha dominant, you may be more likely to develop asthma and other breathing disorders, cancer, diabetes, nausea after eating, and obesity.

To reduce excess Kapha (earth and water) and be more balanced, you can increase the number of fruits and vegetables in your diet and do exercise that gets the blood flowing, like jogging or sun salutations in yoga.

Ayurvedic Treatment

An Ayurvedic practitioner will create a treatment plan specifically designed for you. of treatment, which is to bring your mind and body into balance. They'll take into account your unique physical and emotional makeup and your primary and secondary doshas. They will use that information to work toward the goal.

There are several tools used in Ayurvedic medicine to help you create harmony, avoid disease, and treat conditions you may have. These include:

- Herbal medicine. A key component of Ayurveda is that it's used in different combinations, depending on your dosha, and includes licorice, red clover, ginger, and turmeric.

- Yoga

- Meditation

- Purification programs. Also known as panchakarma, these are used to cleanse your body of undigested food through practices like blood purification, massage, medical oils, herbs, enemas, and laxatives.

- Counseling. Your practitioner will help you understand your dosha, how it impacts your life, and how you can change your lifestyle to create more balance and harmony.

- Other treatments used in Ayurveda include oil massage, breathing exercises (known as pranayama), and repeating mantras or phrases.

It is important to note that the FDA doesn't review or approve ayurvedic products. In fact, it has banned certain ones from entering the country since 2007.

What's more, the FDA has warned that 1 in 5 ayurvedic medicines contain toxic metals like lead, mercury, and arsenic.

These heavy metals can cause life-threatening illnesses, especially in children.

Ayurveda or Ayurvedic medicine is a system of traditional medicine native to India, which uses a range of treatments, including panchakarma ('5 actions'), yoga, massage, acupuncture, and herbal medicine, to encourage health and well-being.

Ayurvedic techniques include:

- dietary changes

- herbal medicine, including combining herbs with metals, minerals, or gems (known as Rasha shastra medicines) that can take the form of pellets, tablets, and powders of various colors and scents)

- acupuncture (practiced by some practitioners)

- massage

- meditation

- breathing exercises

- panchakarma ('5 actions') – a specialized treatment consisting of 5 therapies, including emesis (vomiting), enemas, and blood-letting, which are meant to detoxify the body and balance the doshas (in Ayurveda, the body's three vital energies)

- sound therapy, including the use of mantras

- yoga.

Ayurveda claims to treat a range of disorders.

Ayurveda practitioners believe their approach is effective in treating a range of disorders, including:

- anxiety

- asthma

- arthritis

- digestive problems

- eczema

- high blood pressure

- high cholesterol levels

- rheumatoid arthritis

- stress.

Special considerations – herbs and rasa shastra medicines

Alongside diet, herbal medicine is central to Ayurveda treatment. Safety issues to consider include:

Herbal medicines can be as potent as pharmaceutical drugs and should be treated with the same caution and respect. The belief that herbs are safe and harmless may encourage inappropriate use or overdose.

What is Ayurveda?

Considered by many scholars to be the oldest healing science, Ayurveda is a holistic approach to health designed to help people live long, healthy, balanced lives. The term Ayurveda is taken from the Sanskrit words ayus, meaning life or lifespan, and Veda, meaning knowledge. It has been practiced in India for at least 5,000 years and has recently become popular in Western cultures. The basic principle of Ayurveda is to prevent and treat illness by maintaining balance in the body, mind, and consciousness through proper drinking, diet, and lifestyle, as well as herbal remedies.

How does it work?

According to Ayurvedic beliefs, just as everyone has a unique fingerprint, each person has a distinct pattern of energy, a specific combination of physical, mental, and emotional characteristics. Ayurvedic practitioners also believe there are three basic energy types called doshas, present in every person:

- **Vata**. The energy that controls bodily functions associated with motion, including blood circulation, breathing, blinking, and heartbeat. When Vata's energy is balanced, there is creativity and vitality. Out of balance, vata produces fear and anxiety.

- **Pitta**. Energy controls the body's metabolic systems, including digestion, absorption, nutrition, and temperature. In balance, pitta leads to contentment and intelligence. Out of balance, pitta can cause ulcers and arouse anger.

- **Kapha**. The energy that controls growth in the body. It supplies water to all body parts, moisturizes the skin, and maintains the immune system. In balance, kapha is expressed as love and forgiveness. Out of balance, kapha leads to insecurity and envy.

Ayurveda lowers blood pressure and cholesterol, slows the aging process, and speeds recovery from illness. Many herbs used in Ayurvedic medicine have antioxidant effects, meaning they may help protect against long-term illnesses, such as heart disease and arthritis. Many Ayurvedic practitioners also recommend a vegetarian diet, which is believed to be better for your heart than diets containing red meat.

What should I expect from an Ayurvedic treatment?

Ayurvedic treatment focuses on rebalancing the doshas. On your first visit, the practitioner will take a detailed medical history, check your pulse, feel your abdomen, examine your tongue, eyes, nails, and skin, and listen to the tone of your voice. The practitioner will also ask you questions about your general health, paying special attention to your lifestyle, diet, habits, and surroundings. The practitioner will then recommend ways to restore your natural dosha balance, which almost always includes changes in lifestyle, especially diet. Practitioners draw from more than 20 types of treatment. The most commonly prescribed include:

- **Pranayama.** Breathing exercises. Practicing pranayama helps you feel calm.

- **Abhyanga.** Rubbing the skin with herbal oil increases blood circulation and draws toxins out of the body through the skin.

- **Rasayana.** Using mantras (repeated words or phrases) during meditation combined with certain herbs for rejuvenation.

- **Yoga combines pranayama, movement, and meditation. It has been shown to improve circulation and digestion** and to reduce blood pressure, cholesterol levels, anxiety, and chronic pain.

- **Pancha karma.** Cleansing the body to purify it and reduce cholesterol. Practitioners use methods that cause sweat, bowel movements, and even vomit to cleanse the body of toxins.

- **Herbal medicines.** Prescribing herbs to restore dosha balance.

You must understand the wonderful results of this field of medicine. So, let us discuss some key elements that demonstrate the security and potency of Ayurvedic medications:

Weight Management

Ayurveda supports maintaining a healthy weight following age and height and an optimal body-mass index. Whether you are overweight or underweight, the balanced approach of Ayurveda encourages a healthy metabolism to help you return to your natural weight.

Healthy Skin and Hair

It has been determined that using Ayurveda helps one achieve good mental and physical health and well-being.

This method, which places more emphasis on people than on illnesses, aids in curing diseases and illnesses from the inside out.

Moreover, to comprehend what Ayurveda is and how it works, you must first understand its viewpoints, which indicate that being healthy is your natural condition and that you are unwell if your usual eating habits and surroundings are out of harmony.

Reduces Stress And Anxiety

Research and several studies have found that poor physical health directly impacts how wealthy your mind is. As a result, Ayurveda uses a variety of medicines and treatments to help people reduce worry and stress in their lives.

Those treatment procedures entail yoga, massage, therapies, fasting, and other food restrictions.

Removes Toxins From the Body

Ayurveda says that various kinds of toxins in your body need to be removed. To remove those toxins, multiple treatments, such as Panchakarma therapy, Mud Therapy, Acupuncture, and Shirodhara Treatment, etc., to rejuvenate your body, soul, and mind to the core are offered by multiple ayurvedic hospitals across India.

Improves Immunity And Balance

Ayurveda advises combining a nutritious diet with medicines, proteins, and foods high in proteins to help fight illnesses. Additionally, it supports a stronger immune system and defense system in the body. Moreover, the essential thing is that Ayurveda is not just a system but a lifestyle that you can follow to maintain a healthy balance and boost immunity.

Aids in Weight Management

Even if losing weight is not Ayurveda's main objective, it counts as one of its benefits. Moreover, Ayurveda aids in weight loss without actually harming a person's mental, physical, or emotional health. It encourages weight management through a properly balanced diet, yoga, meditation, stress reduction, etc.

Promotes Digestion

Your digestive system will become stronger as you start eating, and Ayurveda highlights the need to eat certain foods that will activate your digestive system at the appropriate times of the day, resulting in a reduction of toxin buildup in your digestive tract. Additionally, this protects you from feeling tired, makes you feel less irritated, and helps you maintain a healthy weight.

Promotes Self-Love

Amidst the advantages and disadvantages of Ayurvedic medicine, one crucial component of Ayurvedic medicine is that it encourages self-love rather than comparison to others.

Additionally, Ayurveda helps you realize that you are truly unique and have the most individualized path to happiness and health. This indirectly also affects both your healing process and your life by inspiring you to identify your wants and desires. Every person, according to Ayurveda, is a special synthesis of one or more doshas, or forces, known as Vata, Pitta, and Kapha.

Ayurveda, which is interpreted as the "science of long life," is an Indian medical system that dates back at least 5,000 years and is used by doctors and surgeons to promote health and quality of life rather than treat disease. Ayurveda is an exact combination of science and the art of living a healthy lifestyle.

Ayurveda is an ancient science that employs a variety of naturally derived treatments over time. These Ayurvedic therapies are made from plants, natural extracts, and herbs that have been proven to be efficient in treating a range of disorders. The primary goal of ayurvedic therapy is to restore balance to these three major body systems. Ayurveda is a medical system that addresses not only the body but also the mind and spirit. Most diseases associated with psychophysiological and pathologic changes in the body, according to Ayurveda, are caused by an imbalance in three different doshas (i.e., Vata, Pitta, and Kapha).

The side effects of conventional medicine, on the other hand, can range from mild to severe and are all produced in laboratories. Modern medicine is an excellent tool in the treatment of serious illnesses. It is, however, a disease management system, and its function is to manage diseases. When treating an individual, modern medicine must begin to accept and incorporate the mind and emotional aspects of the whole being.

Each person is distinguished by their mind-body type. In Ayurveda, these primary qualities that govern the body are referred to as "doshas."

When these doshas are perfectly balanced, one is in a healthy state. They enter a state of "vikruti" - an imbalanced state of body and mind - when they lose balance due to dehydration, anxiety, stress, low energy, or excessive exertion.

Ayurveda, which is interpreted as the "science of long life," is an Indian medical system that dates back at least 5,000 years and is used by doctors and surgeons to promote health and quality of life rather than treat disease. Ayurveda is an exact combination of science and the art of living a healthy lifestyle.

Ayurveda is an ancient science that employs a variety of naturally derived treatments over time. These Ayurvedic therapies are made from plants, natural extracts, and herbs that have been proven to be efficient in treating a range of disorders. The primary goal of ayurvedic therapy is to restore balance to these three major body systems. Ayurveda is a medical system that addresses not only the body but also the mind and spirit. Most diseases associated with psychophysiological and pathologic changes in the body, according to Ayurveda, are caused by an imbalance in three different doshas (i.e., Vata, Pitta, and Kapha).

The side effects of conventional medicine, on the other hand, can range from mild to severe and are all produced in laboratories. Modern medicine is an excellent tool in the treatment of serious illnesses. It is, however, a disease management system, and its function is to manage diseases. When treating an individual, modern medicine must begin to accept and incorporate the mind and emotional aspects of the whole being.

Benefits of Ayurveda

Ayurveda offers a wide range of therapies and treatments and covers almost every age group.

The following are some of the primary benefits of using Ayurveda on a regular basis.

- Beautiful, healthy skin and hair

- Reduce Stress

- Lower Inflammation

- Weight Management and Loss

- Purify the Body

- Lower blood pressure, cholesterol, and illness and disease symptoms

- Boosts quality of life

- Ayurveda has numerous health-related benefits.

How does Ayurveda medicine work

Ayurveda has described nearly seven different types of inflammation. Ayurvedic medicine considers drugs' behavioral, physiological, and psychological effects on the entire mind-body complex. Ayurvedic treatment begins with internal purification and is followed by a special diet, herbal remedies, massage therapy, yoga, and meditation. The concepts of universal interconnectedness, the body's constitution (Prakriti), and life forces underpin Ayurvedic medicine (doshas).

Each person is distinguished by their mind-body type. In Ayurveda, these primary qualities that govern the body are referred to as "doshas."

When these doshas are perfectly balanced, one is in a healthy state. They enter a state of "vikruti" - an imbalanced state of body and mind - when they lose balance due to dehydration, anxiety, stress, low energy, or excessive exertion.

By balancing the doshas, **Ayurveda** promotes health. Overall, it seeks to maintain and improve overall health, regardless of age.

Long before modern medicine found its way to the far reaches of India, Ayurveda was the primary medical treatment system. Instead of doctors, there were Vaidyas and Rishis who used the knowledge of the Vedas to treat not just minor but major ailments as well. Then, in the 1800s, allopathy made its appearance and paved the way for the medical structure we have today.

Beyond the surface-level differences between Ayurveda and Allopathy, there is a lot more to explore and understand. The different ways both systems work are described below.

What is Ayurveda?

Ayurveda is an alternative holistic medicine system that is one of the oldest of its kind that originated in India. Most modern medicine and treatments find inspiration from Ayurveda.

The Ayurvedic system is all-natural and concentrates on the overall well-being of the human body to treat diseases. It is a system of healing bodies and riding them off ailments by keeping ourselves in balance by eating the right foods and exercising.

Ayurveda categorizes people as a combination of five elements: earth, air, water, space, and fire. These elements work to form three life forces, also called Doshas: Vata, Kapha, and Pitta. A combination of these doshas and elements determines a person's personality and disposition. Ayurvedic doctors also rely on them to prescribe treatment plans.

What is Allopathy?

Allopathy is an umbrella term that refers to all modern and scientific medicines and treatments. All medicines that fall under Allopathy have been clinically tested to ensure that they have no adverse side effects when consumed. The goal of Allopathy is to treat any particular disease with an appropriate medicine that produces an opposite effect on the patient.

With advancements in Medicine, Allopathy is constantly evolving and changing. The term Allopathy is, however, not used as much anymore.

Meaning: -

The word Ayurveda is made up of two words. 'Ayus' means life, and 'Veda' means Science or Intelligence, making Ayurveda 'Intelligence or Knowledge of Life'. On the other hand, the word Allopathy has Greek origins. Firstly, 'állos' means different, and 'pathos' means sickness. Together, it means 'Other than illness'

Focus: -

Ayurveda focuses on naturally curing all diseases of the body. Ayurvedic doctors will focus on not just physical health but mental health, too, using alternative medicine. However, Allopathy is backed by Science. All medicines and treatments used in Allopathy are clinically tested to cure ailments and diseases.

Approach to treatment: -

The approach to Ayurveda is more holistic. Ayurvedic doctors go to the root cause of the problem and then create a plan to remove it.

This treatment includes taking care of mental and physical health. After that, the approach to Allopathy needs to be more holistic. Allopathy doctors will spot-treat diseases and issues. Allopathy aims to provide a quick cure for any given physical disease.

Long-term effect: -

Ayurvedic treatments are more long-term. It is not limited to immediate treatment of any disease and providing quick relief. As stated above, the root cause of the problem will be addressed, and the overall quality of life of the patient will be improved. Allopathy will remove the current problem, but the cure is not permanent. If any further issues arise, they will be approached in the same way. One way of understanding this is in terms of bacteria. Ayurveda will permanently remove the bacteria from the system, while Allopathy will kill the bacteria, but traces of it could remain in the system and crop up later.

Cost: -

Another deciding **difference between Ayurveda and Allopathy** is the cost of both. Ayurveda is significantly lower in cost than Allopathy. One major reason is that Allopathic medicines are Government-regulated, and prices are kept in check. Ayurvedic medicines, however, do not have much Government control. Manufacturers are free to set their prices, and often, they set the prices in the affordable range. The same is true for procedures and treatments for Ayurveda and Allopathy. Ayurvedic treatments are much cheaper, and one does not have to go back for more treatments.

Side Effects and Healing Time: -

Ayurveda is a completely natural method of diagnosing and treating patients. As such, the side effects are minimal, and the positive effects last for a longer time. Due to its nature, Ayurveda takes a long time to heal, as opposed to Allopathy, where the healing time is less, and its effects are felt quicker. Additionally, in Allopathy, the side effects could be more adverse as it involves the use of chemical-based medicines.

The debate of 'Is Ayurveda better than Allopathy' is multifaceted and must be dealt with more easily. Both have their own set of merits, demerits, and a loyal follower base. While Ayurveda can naturally help cure diseases while taking into account the mental and physical state of the patient, Allopathy treatments have been tested and have Scientific backing. When both can help meet the end goal, choosing one would depend on the individual's choices and preferences.

Ayurveda treatment starts with an internal purification process, followed by a special diet, herbal remedies, massage therapy, yoga, and meditation. The concepts of universal interconnectedness, the body's constitution (prakriti), and life forces (doshas) are the primary basis of Ayurvedic medicine.

Ayurveda or Ayurvedic medicine is a system of traditional medicine native to India, which uses a range of treatments, including panchakarma ('5 actions'), yoga, massage, acupuncture, and herbal medicine, to encourage health and wellbeing.

What are the steps in Ayurvedic treatment?

Ayurveda treatment starts with an internal purification process, followed by a special diet, herbal remedies, massage therapy, yoga, and meditation. The concepts of universal interconnectedness, the body's constitution (prakriti), and life forces (doshas) are the primary basis of Ayurvedic medicine.

What are the seven stages of Ayurveda?

In Ayurveda, they are called Sapta Dhatus - Rasa, Rakta, Mamsa, Meda, Asthi, Majja, and Sukhra, respectively.

What is Ayurveda's system approach to health?

Ayurveda has evolved as a holistic system, having an understanding of physiology enabling it to maintain and restore health with a few side effects and will focus rather on health. In contrast, allopathy, whose analytic understanding of physiology leads mainly to the suppression of symptoms with many side effects.

What are the three systems of Ayurveda?

Ayurveda, the traditional medical system of India, has delineated three categories of fundamental regulatory principles of the body, mind, and behavior. These three categories, called doshas, are named Vata, Pitta, and Kapha.

What are the five principles of Ayurveda?

Ayurveda believes that the entire universe is composed of five elements: Vayu (Air), Jala (Water), Aakash (Space or ether), Prithvi (Earth) and Teja (Fire). These five elements (referred to as Pancha Mahabhoota in Ayurveda) are believed to form the three basic humors of the human body in varying combinations.28 Feb 2016

Ayurveda is an ancient Indian system of medicine that aims to promote health and prevent disease by maintaining balance in the body, mind, and spirit. It is based on the concept of three doshas or biological energies, namely Vata, Pitta, and Kapha, which govern all physical and physiological processes in the body. In fact, many treatments in Ayurveda enhance overall well-being. Please find below the six best Ayurveda treatments.

What are the four pillars of life in Ayurveda?

All practitioners would agree on the Four Pillars, but each may have a different order of importance.

THE FOUR PILLARS OF AYURVEDA

- LIFESTYLE: the routine of habits and practices that make up one's day and then flow into weeks, months, and years

- NUTRITION

- SLEEP

- ENERGY/STRESS MANAGEMENT

HOMEOPATHY

Hahnemann conceived of homeopathy while translating a medical treatise by the Scottish physician and chemist William Cullen into German. Being skeptical of Cullen's theory that cinchona cured malaria because it was bitter, Hahnemann ingested some bark specifically to investigate what would happen. He experienced fever, shivering, and joint pain, symptoms similar to those of malaria itself. From this, Hahnemann came to believe that all effective drugs produce symptoms in healthy individuals similar to those of the diseases that they treat. This led to the name *"homeopathy," which comes from the Greek ὅμοιος hómoios, "-like" and πάθος páthos, "suffering."*

The doctrine that those drugs are effective and produce symptoms similar to the symptoms caused by the diseases they treat, called "the law of similars," was expressed by Hahnemann with the Latin phrase *similia similibus curentur*, or "like cures like

As Hahnemann believed that large doses of drugs that caused similar symptoms would only aggravate illness, he advocated for extreme dilutions. A technique was devised for making dilutions that Hahnemann claimed would preserve the substance's therapeutic properties while removing its harmful effects. Hahnemann believed that this process enhanced "the spirit-like medicinal powers of the crude substances." He gathered and published an overview of his new medical system in his book, *The Organon of the Healing Art* (1810), with a sixth edition published in 1921 that homeopaths still use today.

Miasms and disease

In the *Organon*, Hahnemann introduced the concept of "miasms" as the "infectious principles" underlying chronic disease and as "peculiar morbid derangement[s] of vital force." Hahnemann associated each miasm with specific diseases and thought that initial exposure to miasms causes local symptoms, such as skin or venereal diseases. He asserted that if these symptoms were suppressed by medication, the cause went deeper and began to manifest itself as diseases of the internal organs. Homeopathy maintains that treating diseases by directly alleviating their symptoms, as is sometimes done in conventional medicine, is ineffective because all "disease can generally be traced to some latent, deep-seated, underlying chronic, or inherited tendency." The underlying imputed miasm remains, and deep-seated ailments can be corrected only by removing the deeper disturbance of the vital force.

Hahnemann's hypotheses for miasms originally presented only three local symptoms: psora (the itch), syphilis (venereal disease), or sycosis (fig-wart disease). Of these, the most important was psora, which is described as being related to any itching diseases of the skin and is claimed to be the foundation of many further disease conditions. Hahnemann believed it to be the cause of such diseases as epilepsy, cancer, jaundice, deafness, and cataracts. Since Hahnemann's time, other miasms have been proposed, some replacing illnesses previously attributed to the psora, including tuberculosis and cancer miasms.

It was introduced to the United States in 1825 by Hans Birch Gram, a student of Hahnemann. The first homeopathic school in the United States opened in 1835, and the American Institute of Homeopathy was established in 1844. Throughout the 19th century, dozens of homeopathic institutions appeared in Europe and the United States, and by 1900, there were 22 homeopathic colleges and 15,000 practitioners in the United States.

One reason for the growing popularity of homeopathy was its apparent success in treating people suffering from infectious disease epidemics. During 19th-century epidemics of diseases such as cholera, death rates in homeopathic hospitals were often lower than in conventional hospitals, where the treatments used at the time were often harmful and did little or nothing to combat the diseases.

Consultation

Homeopaths generally begin with a consultation, which can be a 10−15 minute appointment or last for over an hour, where the patient describes their medical history. The patient describes the "modalities" or if their symptoms change depending on the weather and other external factors. The practitioner also solicits information on mood, likes and dislikes, physical, mental, and emotional states, life circumstances, and any physical or emotional illnesses. This information (also called the "symptom picture") is matched to the "drug picture" in the *materia medica* or repertory and used to determine the appropriate homeopathic remedies. In classical homeopathy, the practitioner attempts to match a single preparation to the totality of symptoms (the *similar*), while "clinical homeopathy" involves combinations of preparations based on the illness's symptoms.

Homeopathic pills are made from an inert substance (often sugars, typically lactose), upon which a drop of liquid homeopathic preparation is placed and allowed to evaporate.

A more dilute solution is described as having a higher "potency" and thus is claimed to be stronger and deeper-acting. The general method of dilution is serial dilution, where the solvent is added to part of the previous mixture, but the "Korsakovian" method may also be used. In the Korsakovian method, the vessel in which the preparations are manufactured is emptied and refilled with solvent, with the volume of fluid adhering to the walls of the vessel deemed sufficient

As performed by Hahnemann, provings involved administering various preparations to healthy volunteers. The volunteers were then observed, often for months at a time. They were made to keep extensive journals detailing all of their symptoms at specific times throughout the day. They were forbidden from consuming coffee, tea, spices, or wine for the duration of the experiment; playing chess was also prohibited because Hahnemann considered it to be "too exciting," though they were allowed to drink beer and encouraged to exercise in moderation. At first, Hahnemann used undiluted doses for provings, but he later advocated provings with preparations at a 30C dilution, and most modern provings are carried out using ultra-dilute preparations.

Lack of scientific evidence

The lack of convincing scientific evidence supporting its efficacy and its use of preparations without active ingredients have led to characterizations of homeopathy as pseudoscience and quackery, or, in the words of a 1998 medical review, "placebo therapy at best and quackery at worst." The Russian Academy of Sciences considers homeopathy a "dangerous 'pseudoscience' that does not work" and "urges people to treat homeopathy 'on a par with magic.'" The Chief Medical Officer for England, Dame Sally Davies, has stated that homeopathic preparations are "rubbish" and do not serve as anything more than placebos. In 2013, Mark Walport, the UK Government's Chief Scientific Adviser and head of the Government Office for Science, said, "Homeopathy is nonsense; it is non-science." His predecessor, John Beddington, also said that homeopathy "has no underpinning of scientific basis" and is being "fundamentally ignored" by the Government.

Jack Killen, acting deputy director of the National Center for Complementary and Alternative Medicine, says homeopathy "goes beyond current understanding of chemistry and physics." He adds: "There is, to my knowledge, no condition for which homeopathy has been proven to be an effective treatment." Ben Goldacre says that homeopaths who misrepresent scientific evidence to a scientifically illiterate public have "... walled themselves off from academic medicine, and critique has been all too often met with avoidance rather than argument".

In an article entitled "Should We Maintain an Open Mind about Homeopathy?" published in the *American Journal of Medicine*, Michael Baum and Edzard Ernst – writing to other physicians – wrote that "Homeopathy is among the worst examples of faith-based medicine... These axioms [of homeopathy] are not only out of line with scientific facts but also directly opposed to them. If homeopathy is correct, much of physics, chemistry, and pharmacology must be incorrect...".

What Conditions Does Homeopathy Treat?

It's used for a wide variety of health issues, including some chronic illnesses:

- Allergies

- Migraines

- Depression

- Chronic fatigue syndrome

- Rheumatoid arthritis

- Irritable bowel syndrome

- Premenstrual syndrome

It can also be used for minor issues like bruises, scrapes, toothaches, headaches, nausea, coughs, and colds.

Don't use homeopathic medicine for life-threatening illnesses, like asthma, cancer, and heart disease, or in emergencies.

You should also avoid using it in place of vaccines.

- "Like cures like"—the notion that a disease can be cured by a substance that produces similar symptoms in healthy people.

- "Law of minimum dose"—the notion that the lower the dose of the medication, the greater its effectiveness. Many homeopathic products are so diluted that no molecules of the original substance remain.

Homeopathic products come from plants (such as red onion, arnica [mountain herb], poison ivy, belladonna [deadly nightshade], and stinging nettle), minerals (such as white arsenic), or animals (such as crushed whole bees).

Homeopathic products are often made as sugar pellets to be placed under the tongue; they may also be in other forms, such as ointments, gels, drops, creams, and tablets.

Treatments are "individualized" or tailored to each person—it's common for different people with the same condition to receive different treatments.

Homeopathy uses a different diagnostic system for assigning treatments to individuals and recognizes clinical patterns of signs and symptoms that are different from those of conventional medicine.

What should I expect if I try it?

When you first see a homeopath, they'll usually ask you about any specific health conditions and your general well-being, emotional state, lifestyle, and diet.

Based on this, the homeopath decides on the course of treatment, which often involves homeopathic remedies given as pills, capsules, or tinctures (solutions).

Your homeopath may recommend that you attend one or more follow-up appointments so the remedy's effects on your health can be assessed.

When is it used?

Homeopathy is used for an extremely wide range of health conditions. Many practitioners believe it can help with any condition.

Among the most common conditions that people seek homeopathic treatment for are:

- asthma

- ear infections

- hay fever

- mental health conditions, such as depression, stress and anxiety

- allergies, such as food allergies

- dermatitis (an allergic skin condition)

- arthritis

- high blood pressure

There's no good-quality evidence that homeopathy is an effective treatment for these or any other health conditions.

The National Institute for Health and Care Excellence (NICE), which advises the NHS on the use of treatments, doesn't recommend using homeopathy in the treatment of any health condition.

What are the regulation issues?

There's no legal regulation of homeopathic practitioners in the UK. This means that anyone can practice as a homeopath, even if they have no qualifications or experience.

Is homeopathy safe?

Homeopathic remedies are generally safe, and the risk of a serious adverse side effect from taking them is thought to be small. Some homeopathic remedies may contain substances that aren't safe or interfere with the action of other medicines. Herbs and other plants, minerals, venom from snakes, and other substances can be used to make homeopathic remedies. They are diluted again and again and "succussed" or shaken vigorously between each dilution. The process of sequential dilution and succussion is called potentization.

How does homeopathy work?

Homeopathic remedies start with substances, such as herbs, minerals, or animal products. These substances are first crushed and dissolved in a liquid, usually grain, alcohol, or lactose, mechanically shaken and then stored. This is the "mother tincture." Homeopaths then dilute tinctures more with alcohol or lactose, either 1 part to 10 (written as "x") or 1 part to 100 (written as "c"). These tinctures are shaken, yielding a 1x or 1c dilution. Homeopaths can further dilute these tinctures two times (2x or 2c), three times (3x or 3c), and so forth. Many times, professional homeopaths will use much higher dilutions because they believe the more diluted the substance, the more potent its healing powers.

Homeopathic remedies aim to stimulate the body's healing mechanisms. Homeopaths believe that physical disease often has mental and emotional components. Hence, a homeopathic diagnosis includes physical symptoms (such as feverishness), current emotional and psychological state (such as anxiety and restlessness), and the person's constitution. A person's constitution includes qualities related to creativity, initiative, persistence, concentration, physical sensitivities, and stamina. The right remedy for a condition will take all of these aspects into account, so each diagnosis and remedy is individualized. That means three people with hay fever could need three different prescriptions.

Health food stores and some pharmacies sell homeopathic remedies for a variety of problems. Homeopaths often recommend taking remedies for no more than 2 to 3 days, although some people may need only 1 to 2 doses before they start feeling better. In some cases, homeopaths may recommend daily dosing.

What happens during a visit to the homeopath?

Your first visit to the homeopath can take from 1 to 2½ hours. Because homeopaths treat the person rather than the illness, the homeopath will interview you at length, asking many questions and observing personality traits, as well as unusual behavioral and physical symptoms. The homeopath may also perform a physical examination and possibly order laboratory work.

What illnesses and conditions respond well?

Scientific evidence is mixed. In some clinical trials, homeopathy appeared to be no better than a placebo. In other clinical studies, researchers believed they saw benefits from homeopathy. More research is needed.

Preliminary evidence shows that homeopathy may be helpful in treating childhood diarrhea, otitis media (ear infection), asthma, fibromyalgia, chronic fatigue syndrome, symptoms of menopause (such as hot flashes), pain, allergies, upper respiratory tract infections, sore muscles, and colds and flu. Some professional homeopaths specialize in treating serious illnesses, such as cancer, mental illness, and autoimmune diseases. In fact, several studies suggest that homeopathy may have a role in symptom relief and improving the quality of life of cancer patients. You should not treat a life-threatening illness with homeopathy alone. Always make sure that all your healthcare providers know about the therapies you are using.

Homeopathic medicines, because they are diluted, generally do not have side effects. However, some people report feeling worse briefly after starting a homeopathic remedy.

Homeopaths interpret this as the body temporarily stimulating symptoms while it makes an effort to restore health. In people who have serious illnesses, these temporary aggravations of symptoms can be very harmful. Suppose you have a serious physical or mental illness. In that case, you should only use homeopathy under the guidance of a trained practitioner and inform everyone on your healthcare team about any homeopathic medicines you are taking.

Homeopathic medicines that are sufficiently diluted are not known to interfere with conventional drugs. However, if you are currently taking prescription medicines, you should consult your doctor if you are considering using homeopathic remedies.

Is homeopathy regulated?

The U.S. Congress passed a law in 1938 declaring that homeopathic remedies are to be regulated by the U.S. Food and Drug Administration (FDA) in the same manner as nonprescription, over-the-counter (OTC) drugs. This means you can purchase homeopathic medicines without a doctor's prescription. Unlike conventional prescription drugs and new OTC drugs, which must undergo thorough testing and review by the FDA for safety and effectiveness before they can be sold, homeopathic remedies do not have to undergo clinical trials.

Homeopathy also uses the principle of a single remedy, which states that one remedy should cover all the physical, emotional, and mental symptoms of an illness.

Homeopathic medicine is designed to stimulate internal healing mechanisms. Treatments are individualized, and only one medicine is given at a time. Practitioners watch and wait to see if the therapy is working before trying something else.

The reasons for this are that the potential for interactions is unknown, one medicine may cancel the other, and if more than one remedy is taken at a time, it's difficult to tell which one is working.

However, sometimes, a homeopathic treatment will initially aggravate symptoms before showing an improvement. Proponents of homeopathy say a slight worsening of the condition is normal at the beginning and a sign the medicine is prompting the body to heal itself.[2]

Homeopathic remedies are generally safe and without significant side effects since they use only a small amount of a highly diluted substance.

RISING POPULARITY

Thanks to the then-barbaric methods of allopathy, homeopathy caught on like wildfire in Europe and America. Besides royal patronage in European countries, it had renowned proponents like Dickens, Disraeli, Yeats, Thackeray, Goethe, and Pope Pius X. The discipline received a tremendous boost in the 1830s when a cholera epidemic swept Europe. While conventional doctors had a death rate of 50 percent, homeopaths cured 80 percent of their patients. Homeopaths also enjoyed tremendous success in treating cases of yellow fever, typhoid, and scarlet fever.

Homeopathy had a large impact on the practice of medicine. The first homeopathic hospital opened in 1832, and homeopathic medical schools opened all over Europe. Homeopathic hospitals and practitioners often had better outcomes compared to their allopathic counterparts. These improved outcomes were undoubtedly due to the harmful nature of allopathic remedies of the time compared to the non-toxic nature of homeopathic remedies. Thus, the general public began to tout the benefits of homeopathy and demanded better treatment from all physicians.

The new system began taking rapid strides in the New World after Hans Gram, a Dutch homeopath, emigrated to the USA in 1825. In 1844, the American Institute of Homeopathy was formed, America's first national medical society.

Alarmed, conventional doctors formed the American Medical Association (AMA) in 1846. Their primary agenda seemed to halt homeopathy in its tracks. Yet, by 1900, 22 homeopathic colleges, a hundred hospitals, over 1,000 homeopathic pharmacies, and 29 different journals devoted to homeopathy had sprung up in the USA. And nearly 20 percent of doctors were practicing homeopaths.

Between 1829 and 1869, the number of homeopaths in New York doubled every five years. Besides effectively treating infectious diseases, homeopaths provided care for many acute and chronic diseases. Since patients under homeopathic care lived longer, some life insurance companies even offered a 10 percent discount to homeopathic patients! Mark Twain was all praise for the alternative remedy in an 1890 issue of Harper's magazine: "The introduction of homeopathy forced the old school doctor to stir around and learn something of a rational nature about his business." The other advocates included William James, H.W. Longfellow, Nathanial Hawthorne, and Daniel Webster.

By the early part of the twentieth century, homeopathy was in serious decline. The last pure homeopathic medical school in the U.S. closed in 1920, although Hahnemann Medical School in Philadelphia continued to offer homeopathic electives until the 1940s.

Homeopathic practice requires individualization of each treatment, demanding more time than allopathy. This meant that there was more money to be made through allopathy—another blow in the solar plexus for the complementary remedy.

Patients used homeopathy for chronic, physical problems, as well as emotional complaints.[14], [15], [16] The most frequent diagnoses for which they seek homeopathy are allergic rhinitis in adult males, headache in adult females, and atopic dermatitis in children.[17] Homeopathy is one of the most common CAM therapies in cancer care in Europe, ranging from 11% across cancer diagnoses.[18] up to 19% in breast cancer patients[19] Among younger cancer patients in Germany, 45% reported that they had used homeopathic remedies during their illness.[20]

To conclude, homeopathy is likely where the harm is. Although homeopathic remedies do not directly harm patients, it is very possible that harm could occur in homeopathy patients who refrain from seeking traditional medicine.

Patients in the NHS could be indirectly harmed if funds are spent on homeopathy that could have been spent on mainstream care. Patients who are prescribed homeopathic treatments are likely being deceived and, thus, are being treated unethically.

Homeopathy is currently weakening public confidence in the NHS, the MHRA, and science and medicine in general, and also doing a disservice to productive forms of complementary medicine. Most of these unethical effects could be minimized by withdrawing NHS funding for homeopathic practice and educating the public about the lack of an evidence base for homeopathy.

In other words, it would be more ethical for the NHS to stick to treatments of proven worth. There was once a homeopathic hospital in Tunbridge Wells, but it was closed because 'the NHS has to decide the best use of money on the evidence of clinical effectiveness.'[14] Other NHS trusts would do well to follow this example.

STRESS

Stress affects us all. You may notice symptoms of stress when disciplining your kids, during busy times at work, when managing your finances, or when coping with a challenging relationship. Stress is everywhere. And while a little stress is OK -- some stress is actually beneficial -- too much stress can wear you down and make you sick, both mentally and physically.

The first step to controlling stress is knowing its symptoms. But recognizing stress symptoms may be harder than you think. Most of us are so used to being stressed that we often don't know we are stressed until we are at the breaking point.

What Is Stress?

Stress is the body's reaction to harmful situations -- whether they're real or perceived. When you feel threatened, a chemical reaction occurs in your body that allows you to act in a way to prevent injury. This reaction is known as "fight-or-flight" or the stress response. During the stress response, your heart rate increases, breathing quickens, muscles tighten, and blood pressure rises. You've gotten ready to act. It is how you protect yourself.

Stress means different things to different people. What causes stress in one person may be of little concern to another. Some people are better able to handle stress than others. And not all stress is bad. In small doses, stress can help you accomplish tasks and prevent you from getting hurt. For example, stress is what gets you to slam on the brakes to avoid hitting the car in front of you. That's a good thing.

Our bodies are designed to handle small doses of stress. But, we need to be equipped to handle long-term, chronic stress with ill consequences.

What Are the Symptoms of Stress?

Stress can affect all parts of your life, including your emotions, behaviors, thinking ability, and physical health. No part of the body is immune. But, because people handle stress differently, symptoms of stress can vary. Symptoms can be vague and may be the same as those caused by medical conditions. So it is important to discuss them with your doctor. You may have any of the following symptoms of stress.

Emotional symptoms of stress include:

- Becoming easily agitated, frustrated, and moody

- Feeling overwhelmed, as if you are losing control or need to take control

- Having a hard time relaxing and quieting your mind

- Feeling bad about yourself (low self-esteem) and feeling lonely, worthless, and depressed

- Avoiding others

Physical symptoms of stress include:

- Low energy

- Headaches

- Upset stomach, including diarrhea, constipation, and nausea

- Aches, pains, and tense muscles

- Chest pain and rapid heartbeat

- Insomnia

- Frequent colds and infections

- Loss of sexual desire and ability

- Nervousness and shaking, ringing in the ears, and cold or sweaty hands and feet

- Dry mouth and a hard time swallowing

- Clenched jaw and grinding teeth

Cognitive symptoms of stress include:

- Constant worrying

- Racing thoughts

- Forgetfulness and disorganization

- Inability to focus

- Poor judgment

- Being pessimistic or seeing only the negative side

Behavioral symptoms of stress include:

- Changes in appetite -- either not eating or eating too much

- Procrastinating and avoiding responsibilities

- More use of alcohol, drugs, or cigarettes

- Having more nervous behaviors, such as nail biting, fidgeting, and pacing

What Are the Consequences of Long-Term Stress?

A little stress now and then is not something to be concerned about. But ongoing, chronic stress can cause or worsen many serious health problems, including:

- Mental health problems, such as depression, anxiety, and personality disorders

- Cardiovascular disease, including heart disease, high blood pressure, abnormal heart rhythms, heart attacks, and strokes

- Obesity and other eating disorders

- Menstrual problems

- Sexual dysfunction, such as impotence and premature ejaculation in men and loss of sexual desire in men and women

- Skin and hair problems, such as acne, psoriasis, and eczema, and permanent hair loss

- Gastrointestinal problems, such as GERD, gastritis, ulcerative colitis, and irritable colon

Help Is Available for Stress

Stress is a part of life. What matters most is how you handle it. The best thing you can do to prevent stress overload and the health consequences that come with it is to know your stress symptoms.

If you or a loved one is feeling overwhelmed by stress, talk to your doctor. Many symptoms of stress can also be signs of other health problems. Your doctor can evaluate your symptoms and rule out other conditions. If stress is to blame, your doctor can recommend a therapist or counselor to help you better handle your stress.

DISCLAIMER

This book is intended to provide general information and insights into various aspects of wellness, including conventional and alternative treatments, stress management, and the biology of diseases. It is not intended to be a substitute for professional medical advice, diagnosis, or treatment.

The content presented here is based on research, personal experiences, and opinions, and readers are encouraged to consult with qualified healthcare professionals for individualized guidance and recommendations tailored to their specific needs and circumstances.

The author and publisher are not liable for any loss or damage resulting from reliance on the information provided in this book.

Additionally, readers should be aware that the effectiveness and safety of certain treatments may vary depending on individual factors, and it is essential to carefully evaluate all options and make informed decisions regarding healthcare choices.

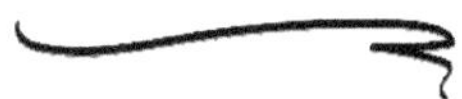

ABOUT ME

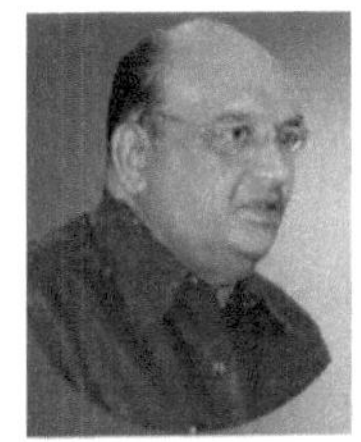 I am **Dr. Prakash Shah**, 79 years old, and I would like to share my short testimony with you. Although I have a longer testimony, I will keep it simple and easy to read. Here are some highlights:

- I draw inspiration from the story of Dronacharya teaching the Pandavas and Kauravas archery. This story taught me the importance of focusing solely on my goals, akin to Arjuna's unwavering focus on the bird's eye. This lesson has shaped my working style, emphasizing the significance of hard work.

- Throughout my schooling, I received blessings from many teachers and principals, maintaining consistently high academic achievements.

- I successfully contested and held various leadership positions in medical associations and social organizations, receiving praise for my work from members and dignitaries alike.

- After completing my MD in Obstetrics and Gynecology, I faced numerous challenges and setbacks before establishing a successful private practice. Despite the difficulties, I persevered with the help of God.

- My interest in Christianity grew after listening to inspiring talks by Joyes Mayer, which provided material for my own speeches during my tenure as a leader in various organizations.

- I have traveled extensively and received training from experts worldwide, contributing to my development as a laparoscopic surgeon and enhancing my medical practice.

- Even during challenging times, such as contracting COVID-19, I relied on my faith and personal treatment methods, ultimately recovering without requiring hospitalization.

- I experienced divine interventions in various situations, such as a kind rickshaw driver returning my lost purse and a stranger helping me at an airport in a time of need.

- Despite facing obstacles, such as the closure of a theology college, I adapted and continued my pursuit of knowledge, eventually obtaining a diploma in theology.

- My life has been filled with miraculous occurrences, demonstrating the presence and assistance of God in every aspect.

My Message to all:

If you pray to God regularly and maintain an honest and helpful attitude, establish a personal relationship with Him, and whenever you are in a dire emergency, God will come without your asking or praying. At such times, God understands your needs and difficulties and will definitely come to your aid. Establish a relationship with God.

Achievements and Awards:

- Practicing Psychiatrist – Psychology – Hypnotherapy
- Training in homeopathy – Ayurveda – Naturopathy - Rackii Medical Professional Contributions – Aroma Therapy - Past Life Therapist
- Obstetrics and Gynaecology Past 30 years in Baroda
- Trained for Laparoscopic Surgery by Upjohn University USA In 1975
- First Laparoscopic Surgeon of Baroda (since 1976)
- Done many Tubectomy Laparoscopic Surgical Camps in Baroda and Broach District (more than 1500 Tubectomy)
- Special recognition as GLORY OF B J MEDICAL COLLEGE at Alumni Conference 2007 Special Training in Various Fields
- Microsurgical Technique of Fallopian Tube Recanalization, British Columbia University, Vancouver, Canada Under Dr Victor Gomel
- Advanced Training in Management of Infertile Couples, John Hopkins University, Baltimore, USA
- Seminar on Advances in Endocrinology in Infertility, Howard Medical School, Boston, USA
- Laparoscopic Surgery In Gynaecology, San Francisco, USA

- Training for Ovarian Hormone and PCOD: Under Dr Stain Leventhal, Boston, USA
- Personalized Training Via Internet - Online in various Alternative Medicine
- Participated in the International Conference of Federation of Obstetrics and Gynaecology Conference, San Francisco, USA
- Fellow and Life Member, American Association of Sex Counsellors, Therapists and Educationists (AASECT)
- President, Indian Medical Association – Baroda Branch, 1985-86
- President, Gujarat State Branch Indian Medical Association, 1985-86
- President, Baroda Obstetrics & Gynaecology Society, 1985-86
- Vice President, Federation of Obstetric & Gynaecological Societies of India
- President, Jain Doctors Federations, Baroda Medical Social Contributions
- Carrier at Lions Clubs International from club presidentship (1988-89) to district governor (1994-95) Raised Rs 43 lacs for sight first projected – Big Event-Film stars and musical – Must Must 94 Night.
- Training to more than 35,000 youths about drug awareness and about sex education

- Numerous projects of Community and social work for down rodents and needy people.

God bless you all.

Yours truly,

Dr. Prakash Shah
Website: www.chronictreat.com
Email: prakashbaroda45@gmail.com
WhatsApp: 9879158791

MAY I ASK YOU FOR A SMALL FAVOR?

First, I want to say a big thanks for reading this book. You could have chosen any other book, but you took mine, and I appreciate this.

I hope you have at least a few actionable insights that will positively impact your daily life.

Can I ask for 30 seconds more of your time?

I'd love it if you could leave a review of the book. That will help me grow my readership by encouraging folks to take a chance on my books.

Keeping it straight - reviews are the lifeblood of any author.

It will take less than a minute of your time but will tremendously help me reach out to more people.

If you liked this book, please consider posting an honest review on your preferred retailer. And I'd love to see your review. Thanks for your support.